The Marlowe Diabetes Library

Good control is in your hands.

Since 1999, Marlowe & Company has established itself as the nation's leading independent publisher of books on diabetes. Now, the Marlowe Diabetes Library, launched in 2007, comprises an ever-expanding list of books on how to thrive while living with diabetes or prediabetes. Authors include world-renowned authorities on diabetes and the glycemic index, medical doctors and research scientists, certified diabetes educators, registered dietitians and other professional clinicians, as well as individuals living and thriving with prediabetes, type 1 or type 2 diabetes. See page 212 for the complete list of Marlowe Diabetes Library titles.

About the Author

DAVID MENDOSA is a freelance journalist and consultant specializing in diabetes. A coauthor of *The New Glucose Revolution: What Makes My Blood Glucose Go Up . . . And Down?*, his articles and columns have appeared in many of the major diabetes magazines and Web sites. He lives in Boulder, Colorado.

Also by David Mendosa

*The New Glucose Revolution: What Makes
My Blood Glucose Go Up . . . And Down?*
(with Jennie Brand-Miller, PhD,
and Kaye Foster-Powell)

LOSING WEIGHT

with Your

DIABETES MEDICATION

How Byetta and Other Drugs
Can Help You Lose More Weight
Than You Ever Thought Possible

DAVID MENDOSA

Foreword by J. Joseph Prendergast, MD

Da Capo
LIFE
LONG

A MEMBER OF THE PERSEUS BOOKS GROUP

Designed by Timm Bryson
Set in 11 point Electra by the Perseus Books Group

Library of Congress Cataloging-in-Publication Data
Mendosa, David.
Losing weight with your diabetes medication : how Byetta and other drugs can help you lose more weight than you ever thought possible / David Mendosa ; foreword by J. Joseph Prendergast. — 1st Da Capo Press ed.
p. cm.
Includes bibliographical references and indexes.
ISBN-13: 978-1-60094-045-3 (alk. paper)
ISBN-10: 1-60094-045-5 (alk. paper)
1. Non-insulin-dependent diabetes. 2. Weight loss. 3. Glucagon-like peptide 1—
Agonists. I. Title.
RC662.18.M46 2007
616.4'62—dc22
2007035614

Published by Da Capo Press
A Member of the Perseus Books Group
www.dacapopress.com

Da Capo Press books are available at special discounts for bulk purchases in the United States by corporations, institutions, and other organizations. For more information, please contact the Special Markets Department at the Perseus Books Group, 2300 Chestnut Street, Suite 200, Philadelphia, PA 19103, or call (800) 255-1514, or e-mail special.markets@perseusbooks.com.

3 4 5 6 7 8 9

Contents

Foreword by J. Joseph Prendergast, MD   *xi*
Introduction   *xvii*

SECTION 1
Diabetes Drugs and Weight

1   **Diabetes and Weight**
     Why Diabetes Doesn't Make You Fat   1

2   **Our Double Bind**
     Which Diabetes Drugs Lead to
     Gaining Weight   7

3   **Byetta's Cousins**
     Other GLP-1 Mimetics
     in Development   17

4   **Other Types of Weight-Loss Drugs**   25

SECTION 2
Byetta

5   **Back When Byetta Began**
     Why a Poisonous Lizard Is
     Good for You   31

6   Byetta's Spectacular Launch   37

7   How GLP-1 Mimetics Work   43

8   Can You Use Byetta?
    The Diabetes Advantage   51

9   Problems with Byetta   59

10   When Byetta Fails   69

SECTION 3
Food

11   The GLP-1 Lifestyle   75

12   The Glycemic and Satiety Indexes   83

13   Spice Up Your Life   91

14   David's Diabetes Diet   95

15   Foods to Avoid   109

16   Sugars   113

17   Bad Fats   119

18   Tips for Weight Loss   125

SECTION 4
Exercise

19   Inefficiency Is NEAT
    Why You Need to Waste Effort   135

20   Aerobic Exercise   139

21   Resistance Is Useful   147

22   Metabolism and Exercise   153

Conclusion   *157*
Endnotes   *163*
Resources   *185*
Glossary   *187*
Acknowledgments   *195*
Index   *197*

*I gratefully dedicate this book to John Dodson
and to Dr. John Eng.*

*John was a major inspiration for me to
start taking Byetta in the first place and he
has become one of my best friends.
Dr. Eng discovered the drug that became Byetta.
These men are my heroes.*

Foreword

By J. Joseph Prendergast, MD

David Mendosa has written an excellent book on *Losing Weight with Your Diabetes Medication: How Byetta and Other Drugs Can Help You Lose More Weight Than You Ever Thought Possible.* This is real-time knowledge about drugs that are revolutionizing diabetes care.

When you first learn that you have diabetes, it is very frightening. A family history might have warned you. You might bring a friend to help absorb the medical advice and treatment plan. You will realize that you face a lifetime vigil, and you will feel that complications are inevitable.

Your doctor will provide technical information tailored to your immediate informational needs. An educational process based on those needs begins.

When you feel comfortable with your level of knowledge, you might look for other mentors, both academic and clinical. Technical information can benefit from real-life common sense. Often, there will be a talented person who will add greatly to your understanding because that person has lived through your experience. Often, this person will be very good at explaining the fine points about diabetes. It might be a writer or a reporter, who can explain all aspects of diabetes care and help you through your life's course. One such person is David Mendosa.

And now we have Byetta and will soon have other drugs in the same class. These are "gut hormones" that mimic how glucagonlike peptide-1 (GLP-1) works. They are given by shot that has been modified to last long enough to enable your pancreas to grow many metabolic cells and, in some people, even to grow insulin-producing beta cells.

David Mendosa explains it well. Byetta is the best new example of why doctors must listen to their patients more than to pharmaceutical marketing and recognize the great potential of new medications. Beta cells that have become prematurely dysfunctional and die prematurely begin to grow back in many people. New "metabolic cells" producing hormones never before known to exist in the company of beta cells may contribute greatly to weight loss. This is very important! There is so much new to learn.

Training of medical professionals in medical school changes over time. Researchers know that learned knowledge must adapt to the power of new observations, as well as information from a patient. The concept of listening to the patient has been the basic tenet of good medical care for as long as I have practiced medicine.

There is a new phenomenon in health care today. Patients are better educated about their medical problems. The Internet has spawned patients' need to know all aspects of their disorder. Doctors today are not surprised by their patients' depth of knowledge about their disease and the range of available treatments.

This has given rise to a new system where the doctors, nurses, medical assistants, and writer/reporters (professionals) need the information of day-to-day observations and conclusions that only patients (amateurs) can provide. This coupling of professional knowledge with the power of patients' important observations is what is called the Professional-Amateur (Pro-Am) joint approach to diabetes care. I first heard this term while reading *The Long Tail* by Chris Anderson, editor in chief of *Wired* magazine. Chris Anderson's business book outlines how this Pro-Am concept is changing every aspect of society, not just diabetes. It is more important today because Byetta has turned diabetes physiology upside down.

David Mendosa's book provides a practical guide to this Pro-Am approach with Byetta. He displays in this book professional and personal experience in the field of diabetes. He has contributed regularly to the field of diabetes care for patients and physicians. This book contributes more.

The book is well buttressed by experience and scientific end notes. Personal interviews with scientists provide key perspectives and information. Mendosa is educating us all about disease and the best treatment.

Mendosa's book explains clearly how these drugs work. He addresses the most important side effect, weight loss. Diets generated by many health professionals have failed to work over time. Though control of food intake is important, a new approach is required.

Weight gain often happens in three stages in those with diabetes. Initially, there is subtle excessive eating. This changes to a subtle increased drive to eat, and ends in out-of-control eating driven by intracellular metabolic changes. This is a phenomenon of diabetes that is often misunderstood. The sequence is powerfully triggered by the insulin resistance of type 2 diabetes. The abnormal intracellular metabolism then contributes to profound fatigue that seems to worsen despite apparent success of conventional therapy.

Insulin resistance can bring on a fear in many patients of diminishing physical capacity or approaching death. Byetta has been important in reversing these symptoms. These patients have a metabolism so totally out of control that it cannot be regulated by conventional therapy. Byetta provides a new powerful treatment we've not had before. No simple nostrum, Byetta. This is metabolic power at its best.

Good control can often mean weight gain. Weight gain seemed to be a certainty of strict control. This is unfair. Often, patients have a technical victory but physically still feel the same. No wonder patients experience a deep frustration.

In chapter 7, Mendosa provides a clear discussion of the role of insulin resistance and in beta cell dysfunction in diabetes and how the Byetta works within these two elements. He gives a good explanation of why aftermeal glucose testing is becoming so important that it may make the A1C disappear from diabetes assessment in the near future. David is ahead of his time.

Mendosa includes an important discussion of the variation of the effect of Byetta in different individuals. This is important for the Pro-Am team to know. He has excellent end notes, just as we would expect from any scholar.

Problems with Byetta are explored. But as Mendosa points out, it would be a shame to give up such a spectacular medication, when most can get a good result with coaching, medication adjustment, determination, and dedication. This is excellent practical advice.

When Byetta fails, it frustrates both the patient and the physician. Deft probing can usually solve the mystery of what allows some people to have spectacular success in their expected parameters while others have only limited success. David reveals his own personal success at overcoming his "plateau."

Mendosa includes the story of the life and times of my Byetta hero, John Dodson. He had personal success at weight loss, reversed his type 2 diabetes, and then completed his quest to get his life back after the death of his wife. Many people have had similar experiences in one form or another. I have learned from all of them.

It is easy to recommend a professional work by someone I so admire. This is an excellent book. I learned a great deal from David's observations. This will benefit my patients with diabetes and enable them to experience the tough spots on their way to success with Byetta. I'm so pleased to be a member of his Pro-Am team. As I have been often heard to say, David, "It's your time."

J. Joseph Prendergast, MD, FACP, FACE
President, Endocrine Metabolic Medical Center
President, Endocrine Therapeutics
President, Pacific Medical Research Foundation
Palo Alto, CA 94306

Introduction

It's easy to lose weight. I've done it hundreds of times. Mark Twain said that about smoking, but he might as well have been talking about losing weight.

Almost everyone who has type 2 diabetes knows about the old weight-loss diets and drugs. Until now, none of them helped us for more than a year or so. Yo-yo dieting even worsens our health. But now we have new drugs for diabetes that help us in new ways, such as making us feel full with less food.

I learned that I had type 2 diabetes in February 1994, when I went to the VA Clinic in Santa Barbara, California, for a pain in my side. After giving me a blood test, a doctor there asked me, "Has anybody ever told you that you have diabetes?" Nobody had even hinted that I might have diabetes. I didn't know the first thing about it. Nobody in my family had diabetes, and I had never met anyone who told me they had it.

MY DIABETES DIAGNOSIS DECISIONS

The diagnosis of diabetes is scary for many people. These people get obsessed with a fear of complications. Other people deny the diagnosis. They act as if they never heard of it. My reaction to my diagnosis of diabetes was different. I was determined to learn everything I could about it. This middle way comes naturally to me because of what I do for a living. I write.

At the time, I wrote for and was an editor of a business magazine. Every time I wrote or edited an article I had to learn something new. It's only news when it's something that you and your readers didn't know before. Learning about diabetes quickly became even more interesting to me than learning about business. As I learned more about diabetes I naturally wanted to share what I learned. Soon, I stopped writing about business so I could write only about diabetes. In 1995, I began to write for diabetes magazines, starting with a review in *Diabetes Interview* about what was then a little-known book about the **glycemic index** that was then only available in Australia. I also began to write articles on the Web, including my own Web site, www.mendosa.com. For the past few years I have written twice-weekly articles about diabetes at www.healthcentral.com/diabetes/c/17. This is my second book dealing with diabetes. Along with Prof. Jennie Brand-Miller and Kaye Foster-Powell, I wrote *The New Glucose Revolution: What Makes My Blood Glucose Go Up . . . And Down?* (2nd edition, Marlowe & Company, 2006). (Note: Terms in **boldface** are defined in the glossary at the end of this book.)

EXERCISING MY FINGERS

Because I am a writer, I spend most of my working hours sitting at a desk in front of a computer monitor. Besides typing as fast as I can, I exercise only my fingers when I work. I was never much of an athlete. My greatest athletic accomplishment came more than a decade before my diabetes diagnosis, when I finished a 10-kilometer race—in the next-to-last position.

Being a writer is an easy life. My life was so easy that I put on more than a few pounds. My lack of exercise and the presence of extra pounds almost certainly had something to do with my diabetes, even if those things didn't directly cause it. So, after the doctor told me that I have diabetes, my first order of business was to take long walks and to begin to lose weight. That worked for a while, but eventually my weight crept up again as I started eating more and stopped taking exercise so seriously.

I HAD TO CHANGE SIZE

After a dozen years with diabetes, I knew I had to make a change. Technically speaking, I was "morbidly obese." My weight may not have been killing me, but it was certainly crippling me. I'm tall—6 foot 2 1/2 inches—but I tipped the scales at 312 pounds and had a **body mass index (BMI)** of 40. I was ashamed that I weighed so much. At the same time, I had almost given up hope that I could ever get down to a normal weight. I knew how to eat low-glycemic food, but I ate too much and exercised too little. A wall of fat separated me from my favorite pastimes. Ever since I was a little boy, I've loved to walk in the woods and hike in the highlands. Being close to the Rocky Mountains is one of the joys of living in Boulder. But a couple of years ago, my doctor told me that the pain in my left knee was arthritis. I could still walk where it was flat, but climbing or coming down hurt too much. Moving my big body became much harder. I had to use a grabber gadget to pick up the newspaper in the driveway. Getting out of an easy chair became more and more of a chore.

I first learned about **Byetta** more than 10 years ago, when it was still called exendin-4. In 2002, I wrote what I think was the first nontechnical article ever about Byetta. This was long before the U.S. Food and Drug Administration, in April 2005, authorized Amylin Pharmaceuticals and Eli Lilly to sell it in the United States.

By February 2006, I was desperate enough to consider taking Byetta myself. There can be negative side effects—especially nausea—but I was still curious. The FDA said that doctors could prescribe Byetta for people with type 2 diabetes who were using the most common drugs for controlling **blood glucose**—one of the **sulfonylureas** or **metformin** or both. (Since then the FDA has said that doctors can prescribe it with some other diabetes drugs, too.) I was taking both a sulfonylurea and metformin when I started on Byetta. My **A1C** level was a bit below 7.0 percent, which some—but not all—diabetes organizations consider adequate.

BYETTA'S POSITIVE SIDE EFFECT

My big interest was in Byetta's positive side effect—weight loss—and less in blood glucose control. But when I studied its prescribing information, I saw that the people in the clinical trials lost only an average of about 6 pounds after 30 weeks. I wasn't impressed. I later spoke with an endocrinologist, Dr. Joe Prendergast, whom I have admired and written about for years.

When he told me about his patients' experiences, I was convinced to try it. Dr. Joe told me that the average weight loss for his 200 patients using Byetta was 35 pounds after nine months. How could his patients be so much more successful in losing weight than those in the clinical trials? I think it was because the people running the clinical trials told them not to change whatever they were doing. But Dr. Joe encouraged his patients to eat less and exercise more, which is precisely what I wanted to do.

I FOUND A DOCTOR

My regular doctor, who had been ragging on me for years to lose weight, didn't know about Byetta. When I asked him to prescribe it for me, he read the clinical trial results but decided I wouldn't lose much weight on it. So I became determined to find a different doctor, and my salvation came in the form of an e-mail from Jeffry N. Gerber, MD, who told me that he is a family doctor who specializes in encouraging his patients to lose weight. His office is south of Denver, almost an hour from my home in Boulder (but a lot closer than Dr. Joe, who practices in California). He wrote that he was eager to start some of his patients on Byetta.

Dr. Jeff wrote, "You can be the first, if you wish." I wished. I wanted better health and knew that my weight was my biggest obstacle. I got my wish for lower weight and better health. Byetta didn't *cause* me to lose weight. But it made losing weight easier. How? By cutting my appetite, so that I was seldom hungry anymore. I totally changed what and how much I ate.

Byetta reduces appetite in two ways. It slows gastric emptying, and it also affects the central nervous system, triggering a feeling of **satiety**. Since I knew that about half of all people who take Byetta have nausea, I prepared for it by eating very little from the first. As a result, I've had almost no negative side effects. The only nausea I experienced was for about three hours when I took the first shot. Once I started injecting Byetta, I began to lose weight immediately. I soon noticed that my trousers and shirts were too loose. I enjoy friends telling me how much thinner I looked.

While lots of things in life are a vicious circle, Byetta and energy are a virtuous circle: The more weight I lost and the more I exercised, the more energy I had. All this feedback gave me more motivation than ever to keep on losing weight. I also noticed that I needed less and less food to fill my stomach as it got smaller.

Since starting on Byetta fewer than two years ago, my weight dropped from 312 to 181 pounds. From the start, I told everyone who would listen that my goal by October 26, 2007, was to weigh less than when the U.S. Army had honorably discharged me 50 years earlier. That meant weighing less than 195 pounds, which would also give me a BMI in the normal range. I have already passed that goal!

With my lower weight, my **blood glucose level** has come way down. My A1C went from 6.8 percent to 4.6 percent, despite my stopping the other diabetes drugs I was taking when I started Byetta. The arthritis that I had is totally gone. I can go for hikes in the highlands again. I also had elevated liver enzymes that showed I had a fatty liver, which can lead to nonalcoholic steatohepatitis and then to liver failure. Now, my liver enzymes are normal. My blood pressure was never all that high, but it, too, has come down. It has dropped from 140 over 80 to about 100 over 60. That's well below the "normal" level of under 120 over 80. All of my cholesterol levels are much better. My total cholesterol has dropped from 225 to 155, well within the normal range of under 200. My LDL cholesterol dropped from 158 to 93, below the recommended level of under 100. My HDL cholesterol—the good stuff—was always far too low. It has gone from 28 to 40, right at the recommended level. My triglycerides went from 193 to 109. That, too, is well within the normal range of up to 150. Now that my weight and blood glucose levels are under control, I feel at least 10 years younger. I have far more energy than I have had in years. Also, my mood is much more positive.

I am such a believer in the company that makes Byetta, Amylin Pharmaceuticals, that about the time I started taking Byetta I bought 100 shares of company's stock. I am still a believer. But I sold my shares later that year, so that what I write won't give even the appearance of a conflict of interest. Sharing what I have learned and experienced about Byetta and losing weight is a lot more important to me than any money I could make as an investor. I offer you this book as encouragement for you to improve your health by losing weight.

MY CLOTHES PROBLEM

The biggest problem is that my waist size dropped from 56 inches to 36 inches. That meant I had to buy a whole new

PROFILE

JOHN MORTENSEN REDUCED HIS A1C

"I think I am pretty typical guy with type 2 diabetes," John Mortensen says. He's a 41-year-old man who got his diabetes diagnosis in his late twenties and has used various medications over the years with differing degrees of success. He says that eight months ago, after a really bad year, his A1C was 9.2. Then, his endocrinologist put him on Byetta. "My blood glucose immediately dropped to where I felt a little light-headed occasionally," he says. While he suffered some of the typical early Byetta side effects such as tummy issues, after a couple of weeks, things leveled out and he began to feel much better. "Then, after three months on the spit, I had lost a good amount of weight, and my A1C was down to an amazing 5.9!"

After some experimentation with Byetta, John says that he has found what works for him. "Basically, I stick to eating around 150 grams of carbs a day," he says. "I think this forces me to choose better foods.

"Byetta's appetite suppression does work for me," John says. "I am rarely hungry. So, now that I am seven months into my Byetta, I have lost more than 60 pounds and am just 20 or so pounds away from a perfect BMI." His latest A1C is an outstanding 5.1. "This stuff changed my life," John exclaims.

wardrobe of slacks, shirts, and underwear, as well as having my ring and watchband resized. At least the size of my feet didn't change! And since my head is still as big as ever, I didn't have to buy any new hats. It turns out that having clothes get too big is a problem I share with lots of people. The launch of Byetta has been so successful that already more than half a million people take it.

My diabetes is under control. It may not be cured, but it certainly is in remission. Now, one problem that I don't have to carry is the invidious label "obese" or "**overweight**." When I reached my original goal of having a normal **BMI,** I began to look ahead. The Harvard Nurses' Health Study showed that a BMI of 23 or below is even healthier, and I have recalibrated my goal to that level. On my frame, that means weighing 181. That's exactly what I weigh as this book goes to press. Having cycled down from "morbidly obese" through "obese," I want a label to describe the new me. We don't have a formal one for it. But about a year ago, I read about a businessman who cares as much about diet and nutrition as making money. The writer described him in a word that stuck in my mind and hope someday people will use when they think of me. That word is trim.

DIABETES AND WEIGHT
Why Diabetes Doesn't Make You Fat

The numbers just don't add up. More than one-third of all American adults are overweight. Plus, nearly one-third of us are obese. Many people think that being heavy causes diabetes. But since a lot more people are overweight or obese than have diabetes, weight can't be its cause. Government data show that 34.1 percent of adults are overweight. These people have a body mass index of 25 to 29.9. Another 32.2 percent are obese, meaning a body mass index of more than 30. Together, almost exactly two-thirds of us are carrying more weight around than is good for our health.

The body mass index, or BMI, is a new term to many people. However, it is the measurement of choice for many physicians and researchers studying weight. BMI uses a formula that takes into account both a person's height and weight. It works well for just about everyone except for children or bodybuilders and others who are unusually muscular. Web sites like nhlbisupport.com/bmi/ make it easy to figure out your BMI, but you can also calculate it without a computer. Here's one way:

> Multiply your weight in pounds by 703.
>
> Divide that answer by your height in inches.
>
> Divide that answer by your height in inches again.

The body mass index isn't perfect. It is a quick and dirty tool that any of us and our doctors can easily and inexpensively use. But it doesn't predict body fat with complete accuracy. That's not the point. The point is that a high BMI is an estimate of body fat measured indirectly. The estimate isn't too good for three groups. For children we need to use a different formula. And for muscular athletes the BMI can lump them into the overweight or obese categories even though most of their extra weight is lean muscle, not fat. Also, some people who score in the healthy BMI area may have a high percentage of body fat and therefore a slightly higher health risk. Nonetheless, if you are an adult who is not particularly athletic, a high BMI needs to be a call to action.

By comparison to the two-thirds of Americans who are overweight or obese with a body mass index of 25 or more, 7 percent of us have diabetes. So being heavy can't be the cause of diabetes. Even when we consider the one-fourth of Americans with prediabetes, there's got to be more to causing diabetes than being well upholstered. Some of the usual suspects include genes and lack of exercise.

Your Link Between Diabetes and Weight

Still, more than 85 percent of people with diabetes are overweight or obese. That means there must be some connection between diabetes and weight. While being overweight can't be the cause of diabetes, weight and diabetes are linked. They probably have a common cause. This strong correlation is why you will often see type 2 diabetes described as a "lifestyle disease." This implies that diabetes results from a choice, just as other lifestyle choices like cigarette smoking and heavy alcohol consumption lead to other diseases. It's blame-the-victim time.

Even the government's Centers for Disease Control and Prevention (CDC) buys into this argument. "We know **obesity** causes about two-thirds of diabetes," the agency told state health agencies in 2005. In fact, no one has ever demonstrated that obesity causes diabetes or even **insulin resistance**. On the other hand, maybe insulin resistance or diabetes makes us overweight. That's certainly possible, but even if it is, something else has to be going on that causes us to carry more weight than we should. Type 2 diabetes generally results from the combination of impaired beta cell function and insulin resistance acting on susceptible genes. Why then is there such a large overlap between being heavy and type 2 diabetes?

The answer is slowly coming out of research led by three scientists who worked together for years in Seattle. They are the endocrinologists Daniel Porte Jr., MD, who is now associated with the VA San Diego Health Care System, and Michael W. Schwartz, now a professor of medicine at the University of Washington; and the psychologist Stephen Woods, now of the department of psychiatry at the University of Cincinnati.

"It's complicated," Dr. Porte says, "because everybody who is obese doesn't have diabetes, and everybody who has diabetes is not obese. So we have been looking at why they tend to overlap."

The answer, they found, is the **beta cells** of the **pancreas** that make and secrete **insulin**. "If the beta cells are not functioning properly this will tend to lead to diabetes," he says. *"And this will also tend toward an increase in body weight."*

Insulin has two apparently contradictory impacts on your body, Dr. Porte says. "One is that it tends to store fat. When you eat a meal, the calories will be stored so that you will be able to survive between meals. But the insulin also goes to your brain to suppress your eating, so you won't overeat."

Obesity too has "a bunch of causes," Dr. Porte says. "Diabetes and obesity occur together more than you would expect by chance." If you have factors in your genes or your environment that would cause obesity, then you would probably become obese, he says, and your diabetes, if any, would be very mild. But if you have factors that tend to damage the beta cells or to produce insulin resistance, then you would get more severe diabetes.

"So you can get varying amounts of diabetes and obesity," he says. "But they will tend to occur together because of the fact that insulin tends to store fat and tells the brain how fat you are, preventing overstorage."

YOUR DIABETES IS BIOLOGICAL, NOT LIFESTYLE

Does this mean that Dr. Porte would not call diabetes or obesity a lifestyle disease? "In our view obesity is not very often a behavioral disorder," he replies. "It is a biological disorder, that is, an interaction between the biology and the environment." While obesity is a biological disorder, he continues, "it is sometime

PROFILE

John Montgomery Downsized

His family and friends say that he has already "downsized" enough, John Montgomery says. But his goal is to lose 10 more pounds. Already, he has gone from 235 pounds to 185 in about 14 months on Byetta. John is 60 and has had type 2 diabetes for about 15 years. "I thought there was no way that the weight would ever come off," he says. "I know that I needed to get the weight down to have a chance to live out a normal life span."

He takes metformin along with the Byetta but stopped taking **Avandia** and a sulfonylurea. His doctor has already cut his blood pressure medicine in half, and he hopes soon to do away with it entirely. John's only negative side effect has been "occasional but significant diarrhea." A positive side effect, he says, is that he is "enjoying a new wardrobe."

amenable to behavioral intervention. But the difficulty occurs when you intervene behaviorally, because that behavior is fighting the biology. That is one of the reasons why it is so hard to regulate your weight. So we need to come up with ways to help people achieve those goals."

This is not to deny that we can control our diabetes better when we lose weight. I know from my experience of losing a lot of weight last year how much better my numbers are and how much better I feel. Now, we have begun to have drugs to help people with diabetes regulate their weight. Maybe in a few years, as more and more of us lose weight, people will stop blaming us for being overweight and stop labeling type 2 diabetes a lifestyle disease.

OUR DOUBLE BIND

Which Diabetes Drugs Lead to Gaining Weight

Almost all of the drugs for controlling type 2 diabetes make us gain weight. In turn, this makes it harder to control diabetes. Most people with diabetes need to take oral medication or insulin to control it. Only 15 percent of us don't take either insulin or oral medication. Since most of the diabetes medicines make us gain weight, we can't win. This is what scientists call a double bind.

YOU ON INSULIN

Until Frederick Banting and Charles Best discovered insulin at the University of Toronto in 1921–22, we didn't have any drugs to help us control our diabetes. Before the discovery of insulin, the only treatment was essentially a starvation diet. In 1921, they successfully extracted insulin from a dog's pancreas. In 1922, Eli Lilly pioneered in introducing the first commercial insulin made from the pancreas of slaughterhouse animals. For 60 years, cattle and pigs were the sources of insulin. Now, however, almost all insulin is synthetic and chemically similar to human insulin.

Before Drs. Banting and Best discovered insulin, people with diabetes were slowly starving and no one with type 1 diabetes would live long. People who began to take insulin quickly gained weight. While that weight gain saved the lives of thousands, if not millions, of people with type 1 diabetes, the weight gain went too far. Like any drug, insulin has its unwanted side effects. One of the side effects of all types and brands of insulin is weight gain.

The United Kingdom Prospective Diabetes Study (UKPDS) is the longest randomized, controlled study ever of people with type 2 diabetes. One part of that study tracked 2,078 people newly diagnosed with type 2 diabetes for six years. This part compared how well they did on insulin, sulfonylureas, and metformin. It turned out that people in two subgroups using insulin gained 22 or 23 pounds in that time. Most of the weight gain came in the first year.

The experience of 9,546 members of Kaiser Permanente Northwest, one of the country's largest health maintenance organizations, is similar. Those who started insulin between 1996 and 2002 and continued to use it for at least a year without adding any other diabetes medication gained an average of 7 pounds.

The medical profession is beginning to recognize this double bind. "Faced with an obese patient with failing glucose control, clinicians must decide whether a further reduction in average glucose level by 10 **mg/dl** to 20 mg/dl is worth another 10 pounds of weight gain," writes Richard Comi, MD. He goes on to note that even the new inhaled insulin is associated with the typical weight gain when people with type 2 diabetes start taking it.

You on Most Orals

We had to wait about 35 years longer for the first oral drug—a pill—to help control diabetes. Orinase (tolbutamide) was the first of the sulfonylurea class of drugs. In 1954, scientists in Germany discovered tolbutamide, and in November 1955, clinical trials began in the United States. By 1957, the Upjohn Company began producing it. We now have about a dozen brands of sulfonylureas plus several combinations with newer drugs. But, like insulin, every one of the sulfonylureas leads to weight gain, although not quite as much as with insulin. People in two subgroups of the UKPDS trial who used a sulfonylurea for six years

---

PROFILE
John Ford had a
Great Round Figure

John Ford is 72 years old and still quite active, he says. "But 14 months ago I was not so active after two knee replacements, operations on four lower back discs, and just plain laziness." He says that he "was able to reach 398 pounds and an equally bright 64-inch waist. Considering round as a figure, I had a very great one."

He was taking 80 units of insulin each night when his doctors introduced him to Byetta. Now he's down to 10 units of insulin each night. His waist is down to 60 inches and his weight is down to 265. "That was my weight when I played football in college."

gained 8 to 12 pounds. Those Kaiser Permanente Northwest members who started a sulfonylurea between 1996 and 2002 and continued to use it for at least a year without adding any other diabetes medication gained an average of 4 pounds.

It wasn't until almost 40 years after the introduction of the first sulfonylurea that the second oral medication became available. In 1995, Bristol-Myers Squibb introduced it as Glucophage. Before then, we didn't have *any* diabetes medication that didn't generally cause us to gain weight. This pill is now also available as generic metformin. People often lose a few pounds on metformin, particularly when they switch from a sulfonylurea. That's one reason why metformin quickly became the biggest-selling pill to help control diabetes. In the UKPDS trial, volunteers who used metformin did lose weight. But it was "a nonsignificant decrease" of 3 pounds in six years, the study authors reported. Those Kaiser Permanente Northwest members who started taking metformin between 1996 and 2002 and continued to use it for at least a year without adding any other diabetes medication lost an average of 5 pounds.

A few years ago, when my endocrinologist suggested that I use metformin, he said that I might lose weight because I would be less hungry. He also warned me to increase my dose gradually so that I could avoid what is delicately called "gastrointestinal distress." More than half of the people have diarrhea and a quarter have nausea when they start taking metformin. I experienced neither less hunger nor gastrointestinal distress. But those are the reasons why many people think that we may lose weight when we take metformin. And I didn't lose any weight either.

In the 1990s, we began to have a much greater choice of pills to help us control our diabetes. In quick succession we got two alpha-glucosidase inhibitors, Precose (acarbose) in 1995 and Glyset (miglitol) in 1996. Neither of these similar drugs will cause you to gain weight, but they won't help you to lose it, either. Both of these drugs are what doctors call "weight neutral." But only a small proportion of people with diabetes take Precose or Glyset, because they are also pretty neutral in reducing blood glucose.

Much more popular are two drugs in yet another class. These drugs are Avandia (rosiglitazone) and Actos (pioglitazone) in the class called the thiazolidinediones, or TZDs for short. The FDA approved both of them in 1999, and both of them lead to weight gain. Those Kaiser Permanente Northwest members who started taking one of the TZDs between 1996 and 2002 and continued to use it for at least a year without adding any other diabetes medication gained an average of 11 pounds, more than those who took insulin and far more than those who took a sulfonylurea. Even more serious is the **meta-analysis** in *The New England Journal of Medicine* that Avandia "significantly increases" the risk of heart attacks. Based on an analysis of 42 studies of the drug, the meta-analysis found that Avandia raises the risk of heart attack by 43 percent and that the increased risk is statistically significant. Dr. Steven Nissen, chief of cardiovascular medicine at the Cleveland Clinic, conducted the meta-analysis, which the *NEJM* published on its Web site on May 21, 2007, ahead of its print publication. The journal's editors do that only with issues that they regard to be of serious public health importance.

Two more drugs to help control blood glucose are **Prandin** (**repaglinide**) of the meglitinide class and **Starlix** (nateglinide), an amino acid derivative. The FDA approved Prandin in 1995 and Starlix in 2000, but both of these drugs also lead to weight gain. In a 24-week clinical trial, the average weight gain for people on Prandin who hadn't previous used a sulfonylurea was 3.3 percent, or 3 pounds. In the Starlix 24-week clinical trial, the average weight gain was 2 pounds more than for those on a **placebo** when they took a 60 mg dose three times a day and 4 pounds more than for those on a placebo when they took a 120 mg dose three times a day.

So, until recently, metformin was the only medication for diabetes that might help you to lose weight. But we now have two exciting options. Like insulin, they are proteins that have to be taken by injection, since stomach acids would deactivate them if we tried to swallow them. But these drugs aren't insulins and they aren't pills. In a sense they are something in between.

YOU ON SYMLIN OR BYETTA

The first of these new drugs to become available was Symlin (pramlintide). In March 2005, the FDA approved this medicine that Amylin Pharmaceuticals developed for people who also take insulin injections. The prescribing information for Symlin shows that people who took it for six months lost about 4 pounds more than those who were taking a placebo in a controlled trial. Symlin might yet prove to be even more effective than Byetta in inducing weight loss. That could be the reason Amylin is working on Symlin more than Byetta as a weight loss

drug for the general population. Its synergy with leptin in rats is impressive,
and it is very likely to be
similar in humans. Symlin
is a man-made version of
the amylin **hormone** that
the body usually makes.
But people who don't have
any or enough natural in-
sulin also don't have any

Symlin helps control blood glucose in three different ways:

1. It helps food move out of the stomach more slowly, which helps control the rate at which glucose enters the blood after you eat.
2. It reduces the amount of glucose that the liver sends into the blood-stream after meals.
3. It decreases the appetite.

or enough amylin. This can increase the swings of your blood
glucose. So, if you take insulin injections, consider taking Symlin, too.

In April 2005, just a month after the FDA approved Symlin,
the agency told Amylin Pharmaceuticals that it could market its
other new diabetes drug, Byetta (**exenatide**). Amylin and Eli
Lilly jointly distribute Byetta in the United States. Eli Lilly
alone distributes it in the European Community. Byetta is a
GLP-1 mimetic. We call them mimetics because they mimic or
imitate the way that human GLP-1 works. Actually, GLP-1
mimetics work even better than our body's own GLP-1, because
they last a lot longer. It is that longer time that is key to how
well they work to control our blood glucose and to keep us from
feeling hungry. Weight loss in the clinical trials of Byetta was
modest. People in the clinical trials lost only an average of
about 6 pounds after 30 weeks. That fact often surprises people,
like me, who take Byetta, since they can experience much
greater weight loss.

You on Januvia

The newest diabetes drug is Januvia (sitagliptin), the first of a new class of diabetes drugs called dipeptidyl peptidase-4 inhibitors. That's so hard to say or spell that people usually just call it a **DPP-4** inhibitor. This class of drugs takes an indirect approach to helping us get the insulin we need from our pancreas only when we need it. Doctors call this getting increased insulin secretion in a glucose-dependent manner. This approach is indirect because it inhibits or restrains the DDP-4 enzyme. That's a good thing, because this enzyme degrades or breaks down GLP-1, something that is key to the subject of this book. Human GLP-1 works for only a few minutes until the DPP-4 enzyme makes it stop working. But DPP-4 drugs like Januvia inhibit the DPP-4 enzyme, so our GLP-1 works longer. One advantage of DPP-4 inhibitors is that we can take them as a pill, rather than as an injection. They help us to control our blood glucose while being weight neutral. DPP-4 inhibitors do not lead to weight loss. GLP-1 mimetics do.

It looks as if the constriction of our double bind is beginning to loosen.

NAME	MANUFACTURER OR U.S. MARKETER	YEAR FDA APPROVED	WEIGHT LOSS EFFECT
Insulin	Eli Lilly, Novo Nordisk, Sanofi-Aventis	1922	Leads to weight gain
Sulfonylureas	Eli Lilly, Pharmacia & Upjohn, Sanofi-Aventis, Pfizer, generic	1957	Leads to weight gain
Glucophage (metformin)	Bristol-Myers Squibb, generic	1995	Possible moderate weight loss
Precose (acarbose)	Bayer	1995	Weight neutral
Glyset (miglitol)	Pharmacia & Upjohn	1996	Weight neutral
Prandin (repaglinide)	Novo Nordisk	1997	Leads to weight gain
Avandia (rosiglitazone)	GlaxoSmithKline	1999	Leads to weight gain
Actos (pioglitazone)	Eli Lilly	1999	Leads to weight gain
Starlix (nateglinide)	Novartis	2000	Leads to weight gain
Symlin (pramlintide)	Amylin	2005	Facilitates weight loss
Byetta (exenatide)	Amylin	2005	Facilitates weight loss
Januvia (sitagliptin)	Merck	2006	Weight neutral

BYETTA'S COUSINS
Other GLP-1 Mimetics in Development

Byetta is making such a difference in the lives of many people with diabetes that lots of pharmaceutical companies around the world are racing to develop similar drugs that will reduce both blood glucose and hunger. Some of these forthcoming drugs have great promise to be more than just "me too" offerings. Nobody is more aware of the competition than the people at Amylin Pharmaceuticals in San Diego, which developed Byetta. They have announced several exciting new prospects.

WOULD YOU LIKE ONE SHOT A WEEK?

Furthest along is Amylin's work with Alkermes and Eli Lilly to develop a long-acting release formulation of Byetta. They call it, at least for now, exenatide LAR. Unlike Byetta, which we need to inject twice a day, the long-acting version will require just a weekly or possibly just a monthly shot. Obviously, this would be more convenient than Byetta. But even more important is that it would work better. That's because the two daily shots of Byetta cover only those two meals, and most of us eat three meals a day. The biggest problem with it is that the two shots don't cover lunch, since you take it only before breakfast and dinner. So it reduces blood glucose levels and hunger after just those meals. The companies developing exenatide LAR started a study in 2006 to see if it is at least as good as Byetta. Elements of this study could eventually form the basis for an FDA submission. Earlier results showed that it reduced blood glucose and weight even more than Byetta does. They plan to ask the FDA to approve it by mid-2009.

Because exenatide LAR works so well, it results in previously unheard-of reductions in blood glucose, according to one of the most impressive **posters** presented at the 66th scientific sessions of the American Diabetes Association in June 2006. It reported on a 15-week study showing an average reduction in A1C of about 1.7 percent among those taking the higher of two trial doses compared with those taking a placebo. That means, for example, that someone who had an unsatisfactory A1C of 8.7 at the beginning of the study would have a good A1C of about 7.0 after less than four months. Those people also lost an average of 8.4 pounds. That's considerably more than people averaged in Byetta's clinical trials over a much longer period. All this with less of the nausea that people on Byetta sometimes experience.

WOULD YOU LIKE TO INHALE BYETTA?

Next in the Amylin pipeline for a drug in the same class as Byetta is a version that can be inhaled rather than injected. That will be great news for anyone with a fear of needles. But it will be difficult, because the drug is a protein, which stomach acids destroy the same way that they generally make injected insulin ineffective. But Exubera, the first inhaled insulin, has proved that the drug companies can make proteins that we can inhale. And in 2006, Amylin started to work with Nastech Pharmaceuticals to develop a nasal formulation of exenatide. A Phase 1 clinical study of this compound began during 2006.

Like many other pharmaceutical companies, Amylin is also working on the combination of two or more drugs that will work together better than any drug might work separately. One such combination joins the hormones pramlintide and leptin. Taking these hormones together resulted in a decrease in food intake and body weight greater than that seen with either hormone separately. Taking leptin also selectively leads to the loss of fat mass and the preservation of lean mass.

LIRAGLUTIDE: THE CHALLENGER IS COMING

Besides Amylin's pipeline for drugs like Byetta, there are many other companies hard at work. Probably furthest along is liraglutide, which earlier bore the name NN2211. The Danish company Novo Nordisk started a Phase 3 clinical trial in February 2006. The company hasn't announced liraglutide's proposed brand name yet but says that it expects to submit liraglutide to the FDA in 2008 and to launch it in 2009. Why such a long wait? People whose job it is to watch the pharmaceutical industry tell me that Novo Nordisk is an exceedingly cautious company. Before it makes a move, it wants to be sure that it has a winner.

The two oral presentations and the three posters about liraglutide at the ADA's June 2006 scientific sessions convinced me that it will be as important for people with type 2 diabetes when it becomes available as Byetta is now. In just 14 weeks, people at the highest dose in one clinical trial ended up with an A1C level 1.74 percent less than those taking a placebo. In the same time period, they lost an average of 6.6 pounds. As with Byetta, some of those taking liraglutide had gastrointestinal side effects. But, as with Byetta, the side effects didn't last. Likewise, liraglutide lowers blood glucose only when levels are too high. So the dangerously low blood glucose levels that we call hypos are unlikely. Unlike Byetta, which requires two injections a day because of its half-life of 2 to 4 hours, liraglutide requires only one daily shot, because it has a much longer half-life, 10 to 18 hours. It gets that longer duration because it binds with **albumin**, a protein that helps to regulate the distribution of water in our body. Binding to albumin renders it resistant to DPP-4.

One of the announcements to come out of the ADA's June 2007 scientific sessions was Novo Nordisk's statement that, like Amylin, it is working on a formulation that can be administered weekly. Novo Nordisk's chief science officer, Mads Krogsgaard Thomsen, said that the company hopes to start Phase 1 testing of it during 2007.

Soon You Will Have Even More Choices

Those are the front-runners. But the race includes many latecomers. PharmaIN, a start-up pharmaceutical company in Seattle, announced at the ADA's June 2007 scientific sessions that it can render human GLP-1, which normally breaks down in a few minutes, long-acting. Its approach is to use a nonimmunogenic nanocarrier that it calls a protected graft copolymer.

A Canadian company called ConjuChem presented data about its GLP-1 mimetic at the ADA's June 2006 scientific sessions. ConjuChem calls its drug CJC-1134 and PC-DAC Exendin-4. It binds with albumin, giving it the long half-life that circulating albumin has. The mice, rats, and monkeys they tested it on had lower A1Cs and weight. ConjuChem has been testing its drug as a once-a-week injection. And a company press release says that clinical trials show that its half-life is even longer than expected so that "an even longer dosing interval may be possible." But a later press release in March 2007 had some bad news for PC-DAC Exendin-4. It doesn't work for weight loss. "There was no statistically significant effect on weight in the treatment cohorts versus baseline or placebo at the end of the 35-day treatment period."

The drug giant GlaxoSmithKline is developing GSK716155 (formerly Albugon). It also uses human albumin. But GSK716155, originally developed by Human Genome Sciences, fuses rather than binds a GLP-1 mimetic with human albumin. It is now in Phase 2 clinical trials.

Another GLP-1 mimetic made it to the ADA's June 2005 scientific sessions, but we have heard very little about it since then. This drug, developed by Eli Lilly, has the decidedly unsexy name LY 548806. But it missed the ADA's June 2006 coming-out event. Maybe that's because Eli Lilly is now working closely with Amylin in marketing Byetta.

Ipsen, a pharmaceutical company headquartered in Paris, is another company with a GLP-1 mimetic. The company reported in June 2006 that this drug, which they call BIM51077, was in Phase 2 trials.

Not everyone working on a GLP-1 mimetic made it to the ADA's June 2005 event in San Diego or its June 2006 event in Washington. Zealand Pharma, based in Copenhagen, developed a GLP-1 mimetic that they called ZP10. Sanofi-Aventis, headquartered in Paris, licensed ZP10 and calls it AVE0010. It is in Phase 2b clinical trials.

Another is BioRexis Pharmaceutical, headquartered in King of Prussia, Pennsylvania. The BioRexis technology fuses GLP-1 with a natural variant of the human blood plasma protein called transferrin. The advantage is that transferrin has a half-life of 14 to 17 days. BioRexis has tested the fusion protein in rats. Its challenge was to keep the potency of GLP-1 and the longer half-life of the blood plasma protein in the fusion protein. The pharmaceutical giant Pfizer seems to think that BioRexis succeeded, since in February 2007 it agreed to buy BioRexis.

Some companies even hope to produce an oral form of GLP-1, avoiding the need to take it by injection. One company that has started talking about oral GLP-1 is Emisphere Technologies in Tarrytown, New York, but their research is still in Phase 1 trials.

CLINICAL TRIALS ARE TRYING TIMES

How far along a drug is in the FDA's clinical trial process makes a huge difference. If a drug company wants to study how its

PROFILE
KAREN D. WANTS TO BE THE
BYETTA POSTER LADY

Karen D., 60, works full time as a nurse while working on an advanced nursing degree. "I don't know if I would have had the energy to do that without Byetta," she told me when I called her. After about a year and a half on Byetta, her weight has stabilized after a loss of more than 50 pounds—her lowest weight in 30 years.

She reports no side effects, except for decreased appetite and easily feeling full. "Satiety is a new experience for me," she exclaims. Sometimes she skips a dose in order to eat dinner, since she is still full from her breakfast dose. "I am so pleased, and I want to be the Byetta poster lady. "Byetta is the best thing since the invention of the wheel, sliced bread, electricity, radio, dishwashers, and microwaves."

Karen has had little stomach distress. Once, when she ate past satiety and did not pay attention to her body, she says that she had one episode of vomiting. Another time, she experienced nausea, because she ate something about an hour before taking Byetta. Now, she avoids eating for two hours before taking her shot, and the episodes never repeated. "My thought," she says, "is that some of the people who complain about nausea are those who nosh all the time."

drug works in humans, the company has to start by submitting an Investigational New Drug application to the FDA. If the FDA agrees, the drug starts Phase 1 testing in humans. At this point, the drug has about a 20 percent chance of reaching the market. And that typically takes five to nine years.

The Phase 1 part of the drug's testing alone takes from one to three years. Then, when it moves into Phase 2 testing, the drug's chance of making it to market improves slightly to just under 30 percent. It then takes about two more years for the Phase 2 trials. Once a drug begins Phase 3 testing it will typically take another three to four years and then has about a 60 percent chance of the FDA's actually approving it. This means that the odds are heavily stacked against any drug in Phase 1 or even Phase 2 testing. That's a good reason not to get too excited about a new drug until it is at least in Phase 3 trials.

When we have at least some of these close and distant cousins to Byetta available for us to use, it will be quite a victory lap for a class of drugs that was unheard-of a few years ago. This will give people with type 2 diabetes some wonderful choices.

OTHER TYPES OF
WEIGHT-LOSS DRUGS

The 7 percent of us in America who have diabetes are lucky compared with the other 59 percent of us who are overweight. Those people can't get a prescription for any of the GLP-1 inhibitors described in the previous chapter unless they can persuade their doctor to prescribe it "off label." That means an unapproved use, which is legal but untested. And even then, it's almost certain that because they don't have diabetes, their health insurance won't cover its cost of about $200 per month. But some other weight-loss drugs are available now, and many more are in the works. You can be sure that the pharmaceutical companies are working as fast as they can to profit from what they call "the obesity epidemic."

Is Alli Your Ally?

In February 2007, the FDA approved the first diet drug that people can buy without a prescription. It is a half-strength version of Roche's Xenical, marketed by GlaxoSmithKline to adults 18 years and older as Alli. Unlike other diet drugs, which work on chemicals in the brain to decrease appetite, Alli and Xenical block the absorption of about a quarter of the fat you eat. The most common side effect is a change in bowel habits, which may include loose stools, the FDA says. People who have had an organ transplant shouldn't take it because of possible drug interactions. In addition, anyone taking blood-thinning medicines or being treated for diabetes or thyroid disease should consult a physician before using Alli. People taking Alli should also take a multivitamin every day, the FDA also says.

A decade ago the FDA approved two drugs for weight loss:

1. The first approved weight-loss drug was sibutramine, in 1997, which Abbott Laboratories markets in North America as Meridia and elsewhere as Reductil. It revs up the **metabolism** and energy levels and also creates a feeling of fullness. It can help you lose a little weight. Typically, in clinical trials, people lost 5 percent of their weight within six months. But like all drugs, it has some unpleasant side effects. In this case, 84 percent of people in clinical trials had higher LDL cholesterol, dry mouth, trouble sleeping, and constipation. Several groups of people need to avoid it, including those who have cardiac risk factors, those who use bronchodilators or take decongestants, and those who use some of the most common types of antidepressants.

2. In 1999, the FDA approved Roche's Xenical (orlistat), which decreases the absorption of fat by about 30 percent. If you have a high-fat diet, it can help. People in clinical trials for a year lost an average of 8 more pounds than those on a placebo. But it can also cause stomach pains, bowel leakage, and diarrhea. It also reduces the amount of fat-soluble vitamins that you need, such as A, D, E, and K, as well as beta-carotene.

You Have Yet More Choices

Other approved weight loss drugs available by prescription are the so-called sympathomimetics. All of them, however, raise blood pressure and heart rate. Doctors can prescribe them for only a few weeks, because they are addictive and because we still have no large-scale, long-term studies of them. They include phentermine, whose names include Lonamin, Oby-Cap, Adipex, Fastin, mazindol, Mazanor, Sanorex, benzphatamine, Didrex, diethylpropion, Tenuate, phendimetrazine, Adipost, Bontril, Melfait, Plegine, Prelu-2, and Statobex.

Some people also use over-the-counter drugs to lose weight. These drugs, such as Dexatrim and Acutrim, primarily contain the active ingredient phenylpropanolamine (PPA). But using diet pills containing PPA will not make a big difference in the rate of weight loss. Recently, spam for Anatrim has bombarded Internet users. The ads describe it as an amazing new diet pill that "makes you crave food less." Some even suggest that Anatrim will improve your mood. If you buy it, it is guaranteed to improve the mood of the people who sell it. Much of the advertising for Anatrim claims that it comes from "Anatrim gordonii," supposedly a South African plant. However, no plant of that name exists in South Africa or anywhere else. Maybe they want us to confuse it with the next nostrum.

That's *Hoodia gordonii*. Some people in South Africa have traditionally used it for its reputed ability to suppress the appetite. And in the United States, it is probably the most widely advertised pill for weight loss. Except that, like Kona coffee, people think they are buying a lot more of it than growers actually produce. And it probably doesn't work. And it may be danger-ous to your liver. And we don't have any proof that hoodia actu-ally suppresses the appetite. And no published peer-reviewed double-blind clinical trials of human use of it show that it's safe or effective.

The world's largest pharmaceutical company, Pfizer, pur-chased and then released the rights to market hoodia. If it worked, why would Pfizer let it go? Most telling to me is what Jasjit Bindra, Pfizer's lead researcher on hoodia, wrote in The *New York Times*: "An early clinical trial indeed showed that hoodia could be a potent appetite suppressant. But there were indica-tions of unwanted effects on the liver caused by other compo-nents, which could not be easily removed from the supplement."

You can also get conjugated linoleic acid—better known as CLA—over the counter. It's a standard at health-food stores. A lot of people buy it, but I'm not sure why. They seem to think that it will reduce body-fat gain and enhance lean body mass. It will help you to trim a bit of body fat, but it has some side ef-fects that you may not want. A recent meta-analysis published in the May 2007 issue of *The American Journal of Clinical Nu-trition* found that people who took 3.2 grams a day of CLA lost almost a pound more in a month that those who got a placebo. But studies found that it can increase the levels of substances in your blood that can put you at greater risk of heart disease.

IN THE PIPELINE FOR YOU

Pfizer is working on other drugs that will help us lose weight. Pfizer says that it has two compounds in the works:

Pfizer's Pipeline

1. The first, CP-945,598, doesn't have much of a name yet. But Pfizer says that people in Phase 2 clinical trials of this cannabinoid receptor blocker have lost up to 8 percent of their body weight within 168 days.
2. Pfizer seems even more excited about another drug candidate, a Microsomal Triglyceride Transfer Protein or MTP blocker. It may lead to the equivalent weight loss in three months as rimonabant (which Sanofi-Aventis subsequently withdrew from the FDA) at six months.

In late 2006, Innodia in Quebec started Phase 2 clinical trials of Adyvia. The company says that taking it leads to weight loss by decreasing the visceral fat that surrounds organs like the liver and kidneys.

How would you like to just spray something in your nose that would stop you from eating too much by blocking your senses of smell and taste? An early stage biopharmaceutical company in Boston, Compellis Pharmaceuticals, has a patent for its CP404 that it says will do that. However, before we can actually use the stuff, the company has to complete clinical trials, which will take several years.

Orexigen Therapeutics in San Diego is a start-up biopharmaceutical firm working on central nervous system regulation of appetite and energy expenditure. The company is testing drug combinations that it expects will generate weight loss and limit the effect of the pathways in the brain that make it difficult for people to maintain weight loss. Orexigen is working on drug combinations. Its lead combinations are Contrave, which has completed Phase 2 trials, and Excalia, which has completed Phase 1 testing. Contrave is a fixed-dose combination of naltrexone SR and bupropion SR. Excalia is a fixed-dose combination of zonisamide SR and bupropion SR. Phase 2 testing results showed that, in 24 weeks, people lost an average of 8.8 percent more on Excalia than those on a placebo. However, it could take four or more years for Excalia to become available.

Manhattan Pharmaceuticals in New York City has completed Phase 2 clinical trials of the synthetic form of oleoylestrone or OE for short. OE is a molecule that exists naturally in the body. Like Byetta, it seems to act on the hypothalamus to reset the body's food control center. But OE also leads to reduced fat storage and allows muscles to use fat as an alternative energy source. In preclinical animal studies, OE resulted in significant weight loss. A most promising result was that the treated animals maintained their fat loss even after they stopped getting OE. Manhattan Pharmaceuticals licensed OE from researchers at the University of Barcelona in Spain, including Dr. Maria Alemany, who was morbidly obese but lost substantial weight when he tested OE on himself.

Pharmaceutical and biotechnology companies around the world are certainly working as fast as they can to develop any sort of magic tablet to help us lose weight. I don't think any question remains that some day we will have a wide choice.

BACK WHEN BYETTA BEGAN

Why a Poisonous Lizard Is Good for You

Some people who take Byetta fondly call it Lizzie or lizard spit and call themselves lizard lovers. They are referring to a poisonous lizard called the **Gila monster**, which produces a long-acting mimetic of the GLP-1 that we have in our bodies.

The Gila (pronounced HEE-la) monster and the closely related Mexican beaded lizard are the only known venomous lizards in the world. In the wild, the Gila monster lives in the American Southwest and northern Mexico. The Gila monster is the largest native American lizard, but you won't see it in the wild much. For one thing, it spends more than 90 percent of its time burrowed underground. For another, it is a vulnerable species likely to become endangered, although Arizona state law gives it some protection. Gila monsters have an even bigger problem with food than we do. Their diet is less varied than ours. They like to eat small rodents, baby birds, and the eggs of birds and reptiles. But this diet is hard to find in the desert where the Gila monster lives. So an adult Gila monster eats everything it needs for a whole year in just three or four meals.

How does a Gila monster survive? If we ate only once a season, our blood glucose level would drop far too low after just a day or two. Recently, scientists discovered the lizard's secret of survival. That secret is something similar to the GLP-1 that we have in our bodies. But it keeps working a lot longer.

DR. ENG'S IRONIC DISCOVERY

In April 2002, when I first interviewed the doctor who discovered Byetta, he told me that he had never seen a Gila monster. That's one of the many ironies in the story of Byetta's discovery. The doctor who discovered Byetta is an endocrinologist named John Eng. Dr. Eng has worked all his professional life at the Veterans Affairs (formerly Adminstration) Medical Center in the Bronx, in New York City. By the time I talked to Dr. Eng the second time, in October 2006, he had seen a Gila monster. "I finally saw one a couple of years ago," he told me. At that time he was in a film shown on public television that British wildlife experts had made. I got a chance to see two Gila monsters myself in November 2006. The American Museum of Natural History in New York featured them in a display of live lizards. They may be venomous, but they are beautiful in their own wild way and certainly in the way they work.

In the 1980s, Dr. Eng was a researcher trying to develop a new type of chemical assay. For years he had worked with his mentor, Dr. Rosalyn S. Yalow, who won the 1977 Nobel Prize in Physiology or Medicine for developing radioimmunoassays of **peptide hormones**. The first hormones discovered were those in the greatest abundance, like insulin. Dr. Eng began by using radioimmunoassays.

"It is easy to detect hormones with radioimmunoassays," he recalls. "But the disadvantage of using them is that you detect what the assay was developed for. It isn't a good way to discover new hormones." And like his mentor, Dr. Eng wanted to discover new hormones. "In research, we always want to find something new," he told me. "And I am no exception. The history of endocrinology is the discovery of hormones."

So Dr. Eng turned to what was then a new way to discover previously unknown hormones. He started to look for them with a chemical assay. About the time that Dr. Eng started his professional career, researchers at Sweden's Karolinska Institute described how they had found this new way to look for peptide hormones. Dr. Eng remembers how exciting those papers were to him. The Swedish scientists "had a well-developed assay, and it didn't make sense for me to try to emulate them," he continued. **Peptides** are chains of amino acids. One end of the chain is the C-terminal amide. The Swedish scientists discovered many new hormones by looking at this end of the chain. But what about the other end of the chain, the N-terminal end? Dr. Eng said to himself that if the amino acid histidine was at that terminal, it would mark it as a candidate hormone.

"That was the concept," he told me. "Now I had to prove it." He started by making it easy for himself, working with a known hormone. "You want to stack things on your side." So he looked at **glucagon**, which the pancreas produces in abundance. "It was so easy that it wasn't fair." Then, he took a more difficult step. Other researchers had reported that they found a hormone in the saliva of poisonous lizards. So Dr. Eng resolved that this would be the next test to put the chemical assay to. The breakthrough came as he looked for histidine at the N-terminal end. "And I found two peaks among the fractions," he told me. "One very large one and one small one. My thought was that the very large one was what the other researchers had recorded." But it wasn't. It gave a sequence never before described. Until that moment the large peak had been completely unknown.

His discovery posed a number of questions for Dr. Eng. The first was what to call it. He named it exendin. "I tried to give it some significance." *Ex* stands for *ex*ocrine, an external secretion. Saliva is an exocrine secretion. Then, *end* and *in* stand for the *end*ocrine function that this external secretion has. The next question facing Dr. Eng was much harder and considerably more important. "I had to show that it had biological activity. Otherwise, it's just another peptide." In a series of journal articles starting in 1990 he set forth his proof of its biological activity and that exendin acts on the GLP-1 receptor. *The Journal of Biological Chemistry* published his initial findings. His first article on exendin from the Gila monster came out in the April 15, 1992, issue of *The Journal of Biological Chemistry*.

Dr. Eng first discovered exendin in the saliva of the Mexican beaded lizard, which has the descriptive scientific name *Heloderma horridum*. He named it exendin-3. But this hormone was vasoactive, which means that it contracts or dilates blood vessels. That prompted him to look at Gila monster saliva, which is not vasoactive. There, in the lizard with the scientific name

Heloderma suspectum, he discovered exendin-4. It is similar in structure to human GLP-1, which slows gastric emptying and stimulates the secretion of insulin, but only when our blood glucose level is high. Exendin-4 has a huge advantage over the GLP-1 that our bodies produce. It keeps working for 12 hours or more to control our blood glucose levels and keep our hunger in check. Human GLP-1, on the other hand, stops working in a matter of minutes. That means that the only way we could use it to lose a lot of weight would be with a continuous infusion drip. Not fun.

So Dr. Eng tried to get the U.S. Department of Veterans Affairs, where he has spent his entire career, to patent his invention. But at that time the VA was only interested in patenting inventions that were specific to the problems of veterans, such as spinal cord injury, loss of limbs, or prostheses. "That put me in a difficult position," he told me, "because it meant I had to essentially make a bet. Patenting it came out of my pocket with no guarantee that anything would come of it. But exendin-4 required patent protection before any pharmaceutical company would risk hundreds of millions of dollars to develop it." He filed his patent application in 1993. Two years later, on June 13, 1995, the United States Patent and Trademark Office issued patent 5,424,286 to him.

Then, he tried to interest the drug companies. At Eli Lilly, he met with people in chemistry, manufacturing, and physiology all day long for a half hour each. "It was like a job interview." They turned him down. Frustrated by his lack of success in finding a company that would try to develop exendin-4, he decided to present a poster at the annual meeting of the American Diabetes Association. In September 1996, he went to San Francisco and tried to find someone to listen to his presentation.

AMYLIN WAS AWAKE

Someone did. He was Andrew Young, then the head of physiology for Amylin Pharmaceuticals and now Amylin's vice president and senior research fellow. Dr. Young saw immediately what exendin-4 could do and called a meeting of the company's top officers. Within a month, Dr. Eng licensed his discovery to Amylin. But it was a rocky road for the small start-up company. By October 1998, Amylin's stock had tanked at 34 cents, and to keep going, the company cut its staff from 300 to 37.

All along the way, the Byetta story has been full of ironies. One was the fact that while Eli Lilly turned down the chance to develop what became Byetta, it was the company that Amylin turned to in order to jointly market it. In 2002, Lilly and Amylin worked out a $325 million deal. One of the strangest ironies is that none of Dr. Eng's research articles or his patent on extendin even mention the weight loss that it often leads to. I asked him in October 2006 when it was that he realized it could lead to weight loss. "I didn't," he replied. It was only in Amylin's Phase 3 trials that the weight loss became apparent, he told me. Finally, Dr. Eng told me that he hasn't been able to prescribe Byetta. He can't, because it isn't in the VA formulary. "That's ironic," he says.

BYETTA'S
SPECTACULAR LAUNCH

Compared to the 13 years that it took for Byetta become available for us to use, its trajectory since the FDA approved it, on April 28, 2005, seems unbelievably rapid. Dr. John Eng's first report on exendin from the Gila monster—which in synthesized form is now Byetta—appeared on April 15, 1992. It wasn't until June 2005 that pharmacies began to have Byetta available. What took them so long?

Basically, the answer is that it took years of more and more testing. And in fact, the 13 years it took from discovery to approval is but the blink of an eye in terms of normal drug discovery and availability. Take, for example, the world's most common drug, aspirin. It was 2,400 years ago that Hippocrates, the father of medicine, told the world that the powder made from the bark and leaves of the willow tree helped to heal headaches, pains, and fevers. But only in 1829 did researchers discover that it was the salicin in willow plants that gives us pain relief. And it wasn't until 1915 that a German company called Bayer sold the first aspirin tablets. It took that long for aspirin to come to market—and that was even before the U.S. Congress required that the FDA approve all new drugs before we could use them.

BYETTA'S TAKEOFF

So Byetta's development was relatively quick. Even more so was its takeoff once it hit the market. Nobody was prepared for it. Certainly not Amylin Pharmaceuticals, although the whole company believed in Byetta so much that they continued to test it even as the company itself threatened to go under from lack of cash flow. And not even Eli Lilly, which came to Amylin's rescue with a huge cash infusion, was prepared. The people at these companies knew they had a good thing. But they still had no idea how good a thing they had.

The first people to take Byetta told their friends and associates about how well it controlled their blood glucose levels and their weight. Their friends and associates could see for themselves how well the weight loss worked. This word of mouth is the most effective marketing tool, but for a while it turned out to be almost too effective. Byetta had one of the fastest takeoffs of any drugs in the history of diabetes. But just a year after Byetta hit the market, Amylin and Lilly had to tell doctors to stop writing new prescriptions for it. They were simply powerless to keep up with demand.

BYETTA'S SHORTAGE SETBACK

The companies had to ask doctors to hold off on prescribing Byetta to new patients so that people who were already relying on it would still to be able to get it. The problem was a shortage of the pen cartridges, not the drug itself. The British company that made them couldn't keep up. Eli Lilly assembles and manufactures the pens, but not the cartridge inside of the pen. A British company called Wockhart UK that made the cartridges wasn't able to keep up with the demand. Eventually, they enlisted an American company, Baxter Pharmaceuticals, to begin producing enough of the cartridges to meet the great demand for Byetta. The shortage temporarily drove down Amylin's stock price, which tells me that some investors were in it strictly for the short term. This speculator mentality doesn't make me happy, because at that time I owned some of Amylin's stock.

PROFILE
RENEE GERGER DOESN'T LOOK FOR FOOD ALL THE TIME

In her first six months of taking Byetta, Renee tells me, she lost 30 pounds. Her goal is to lose another 20 pounds. But she won't tell me how much she weighs.

"I laughed when I heard your question," she says. "I said to my husband, 'Only a man could expect a woman to discuss actual numbers.'"

Even with her weight loss so far, her blood glucose levels weren't low enough. Then, her doctor added Starlix, which she takes just before meals. She says that now her levels are excellent and she continues to lose weight.

"I am delighted with the results of taking Byetta and with the wonderful feeling of not looking for food all the time," she says. "As a matter of fact, sometimes it is difficult to eat enough, because food just does not appeal to me some of the time."

Since then, however, I sold that stock, because I didn't want anybody to think that I was a shill for Amylin.

THE STAR OF THE SHOW

The best and most concentrated publicity that Byetta ever got came in June 2006 in Washington, D.C. There, the American Diabetes Association held its 66th annual scientific sessions. Byetta was the star of the show. Byetta generated huge excitement among many of the 17,000 to 18,000 endocrinologists and other diabetes professionals who came from around the world to attend the ADA convention. The biggest presentations there drew crowds of about 1,000 people each on June 10 and June 11 to listen to experts discuss Byetta and its cousins. I crowded in to listen to those and other presentations. Altogether, 17 oral and poster presentations dealt with exenatide, the generic name for Byetta, in the 2006 scientific sessions, up from seven in 2005.

"From November to January, monthly prescriptions rose almost 40 percent," Alex Berenson wrote in The New York Times on March 2, 2006. By the end of 2006, Ginger Graham, who was then the chief executive officer of Amylin Pharmaceuticals, estimated that more than half a million people were using Byetta. The biggest problem that the company had in the first year and a half that Byetta was available was the necessary halt in writing new prescriptions. There could be worse problems.

More recently, 8 percent of health care professionals polled at the 3rd Annual Clinical Diabetes Technology meeting in April 2007 in San Diego said that they currently use Byetta as initial therapy for their type 2 patients. That relatively low proportion is probably because many health insurance plans will approve Byetta only as an add-on therapy. By contrast, 36 percent said it would be their therapy of choice if they themselves were diagnosed.

HOW GLP-1
MIMETICS WORK

The unique thing about these drugs that mimic our **glucagon-like peptide-1** (GLP-1) is that they work in so many ways to help us control our diabetes. Older drugs like the sulfonylureas help the body release more insulin. Metformin, Avandia, and Actos make the insulin that the body produces work better. Precose and Glyset delay the digestion of sugars and starches.

Type 2 diabetes results from two separate problems:

1. Beta cell dysfunction. Our beta cells don't work as well as they should—they don't secrete enough insulin—or we have lost too many of them.
2. Insulin resistance. The cells of our body no longer respond well to insulin or use it properly. As a result, the beta cells send more insulin into the bloodstream in an effort to reduce blood glucose levels.

Byetta and the other GLP-1 mimetics copy the way GLP-1 works—except that they work a lot longer than the few minutes that the natural GLP-1 in our bodies works. So these drugs do at least six things for us. And they do them all well:

1. Byetta and other GLP-1 mimetics stimulate the secretion of insulin, but only when our blood glucose level is high. This means that these GLP-1 mimetics themselves won't cause dangerous drops in blood glucose, the way insulin and the sulfonylureas can. Some people therefore call them "smart drugs."

2. These GLP-1 mimetics stop the liver from making too much glucose when your body doesn't need it, especially after meals.

3. These GLP-1 mimetics restore the release of insulin in the first 10 minutes after eating starches or sugars. People who have type 2 diabetes have generally lost this "first-phase insulin response" that people who don't have diabetes have.

4. At least in animal experiments so far, Byetta and possibly other GLP-1 mimetics will stimulate the birth of new beta cells, make more beta cells develop, and increase the mass of beta cells. And in test tube experiments, these drugs prevent or slow the death of beta cells.

5. These GLP-1 mimetics slow digestion. Slower gastric emptying allows insulin secretion and nutrient delivery to occur closer together. This leads, in turn, to lower blood glucose levels after eating.

6. And—directly relevant to the subject of this book—these GLP-1 mimetics reduce our appetite. They affect the central nervous system, triggering a feeling of satiety.

I can think of three ways that something could make us less hungry—physically, mentally, and spiritually. As far as I know, spiritual ways, such as blessing Byetta or the other GLP-1 mimetics or praying over them, haven't been tested. But these drugs certainly do work in the other two ways. The physical way is the slowing of food leaving our stomachs so we stay fuller longer. Mentally, the GLP-1 mimetics bind to receptors in the hypothalamus portion of our brains to promote satiety.

The end result of these effects is that most people who use Byetta now and those who, we hope, will be able to use the other GLP-1 mimetics when they become available will have significantly lower blood glucose levels. Most people who use these drugs will lose weight, as well, although it will be considered just a side effect. While scientists are still testing the other GLP-1 mimetics, they seem to have the same effect of lower blood glucose and the side effect of losing weight.

How You Take It

Byetta comes in something like a thick pen containing a cartridge. In the cartridge is a premeasured dose of the drug. This is similar to the insulin pens that more and more people who rely on insulin use because of their greater convenience than the traditional vial and syringe. But a Byetta pen is easier to use than one for insulin because of its prefilled pen design and simple dosing schedule. Unlike insulin pens, for which you have to decide how much to take and to twist a dial before injecting it, the Byetta dose is either 5 mcg or 10 mcg, depending on which pen you use. Typically, when you start on Byetta, you start with the 5 mcg dose for a month or two. Then you go to the 10 mcg dose. You take Byetta at any time from just before eating to up to an hour before the meal. And you don't eat for an hour or two before taking it. You take the two daily shots about 6 or more hours apart. You take the shots in your stomach, upper leg, or upper arm. Personally, I started taking the shots in my stomach and never tried the other sites. I take the morning shot on the right side of my stomach and the evening shot on the left side.

PROFILE
Jim Coliton Stopped Byetta

Jim Coliton started Byetta in September 2005 and stopped taking it in April 2006 because he no longer needed it to control his diabetes. During that time, his monthly average weight fell from 267 pounds to 211 pounds. His goal is to get down to around 205, and he expects to be there soon. He had been losing weight before he started Byetta, so the weight loss is not solely due to Byetta, he says.

Jim is 46 and was diagnosed with diabetes in 1992. For about 13 years before he discovered Byetta, he took a variety of oral medications for diabetes, high cholesterol, and high blood pressure. "Byetta was the last diabetes medicine I needed to take," he says. "When I was able to discontinue the Byetta, I was able to totally control my diabetes through diet and exercise. I am also off my cholesterol meds and control that through diet as well." He has also cut back on but not yet stopped his blood pressure medication. His most recent A1C was 5.4.

"When I was actively part of the Byetta community (I have not kept up with recent developments since I stopped using it)," Jim

Based on the experience that we have of checking our blood glucose levels with fingerstick tests, many of us are surprised at the lack of pain from injecting Byetta. The difference is simply that the places we inject have far fewer nerve endings than our fingertips do. But I know from experience that my stomach does have a nerve ending or two every square inch or so. Sometimes I hit one, reminding me of the daily drill of checking my blood glucose on my fingertips. Here, my wife's experience of years of taking insulin was most helpful. She suggested that

wrote me, "there was no specific evidence that Byetta helped cure diabetes by promoting healthy beta cells. I know that for me the hope of a cure was an important part of my own recovery from diabetes. I do not think of myself as cured, but I am totally diet and exercise controlled and have not needed any medicine for over a year. I still check my blood sugar about once a week and it runs in the 80–95 range fasting."

Jim dieted on and off for most of his adult life. He lost about 60 pounds in high school and put it back on within a couple of years. Later, he joined Weight Watchers four times and had some success but never kept the weight off.

What worked for Jim was reducing his portion sizes, eating more protein and fewer carbs, and closely monitoring his blood glucose and weight. What he finds amazing is the tight control over his blood glucose during the time he used Byetta. "Before starting the Byetta, I had an average range of 30–40 points in a day, testing three times a day, before meals. After I started Byetta, I was also testing in the evening postprandial, and my average daily spread fell to about 15–20 points. My life has changed," he concludes, "and Byetta was an important part of that change."

before picking the exact place to inject, just touch the pen needle to the skin. If you feel anything, move elsewhere.

Since Byetta stimulates the beta cells of the pancreas to release insulin only when your blood glucose is high, the time to take it is before eating. That's why you take it any time from just before breakfast and dinner to up to an hour before those meals.

Working after Meals for You

But this means Byetta isn't working for you all the time. You can't rely on Byetta to directly control blood glucose levels before breakfast. How important is the fact that Byetta works only after a meal? It depends. If you have your diabetes under good control, Byetta will only make that control better. But if your control isn't so good, Byetta won't help nearly as much. What we mean by good control is subjective. But researchers often use an A1C level of 7.0 as the dividing line. It's what three French scientists, led by Louis Monnier, MD, used in their research.

When you have high blood glucose levels after meals, this high postprandial level has a greater effect on your A1C levels than if your diabetes were under good control. Dr. Monnier's group found that when our A1C results are less than 7.0, mealtime glucose contributes about 70 percent of the A1C. However, when your A1C results are high—greater than 10.2 percent—it is instead your fasting blood glucose that contributes 70 percent of your A1C value. This means that Byetta starts working even better for you once you start bringing your blood glucose levels under better control. The better your levels, the more you can keep improving them with Byetta. I experienced this myself. At first, my A1C level dropped slowly, but then the decrease speeded up.

In the introduction I discussed how losing weight on Byetta gives us more energy, which leads us to get more exercise, which, in turn, gives us even more energy. This is the opposite of the vicious circle that is the way that much of the world works. The way GLP-1 mimetics like Byetta work to bring your blood glucose levels under better control as those levels drop is another example of their virtuous circle.

CAN YOU USE BYETTA?

The Diabetes Advantage

You don't have to have diabetes to take Byetta, but it sure helps. Byetta will help most people to lose weight. But unless you have diabetes, it's unlikely, if not impossible, that you will be able to persuade your insurance company to pay for it. Without insurance, Byetta is expensive. The best price I have been able to find for a regular 10 mcg pen is more than $200. This is for just one month.

That's not the only problem that people who don't have diabetes will face in getting Byetta. The other big problem will be to find a doctor who will prescribe it. The FDA has approved it only for people with diabetes. Doctors may legally prescribe it to people who don't have diabetes, but that is considered an "off-label" use that many doctors are reluctant to prescribe.

YOU ARE LUCKY TO HAVE TYPE 2

Not only do you generally have to have diabetes to get Byetta, you specifically have to have type 2 diabetes. It seems that your body has to produce at least some insulin for it to work for you. The 5 or 10 percent of people with diabetes who have the type 1 condition won't benefit from it. Fortunately, most people with type 1 diabetes are thin, so they don't need it anyway, at least for weight loss.

Byetta is theoretically just for helping people with type 2 diabetes to bring down their blood glucose levels and not really for

PROFILE
CAT ALLARD CAN'T GET INSURANCE COVERAGE FOR BYETTA

When Cat Allard started talking the 10 mcg Byetta dose, it made him a bit sick to his stomach. Not every time, but often enough that it was inconvenient. So he went back to the 5 mcg dose, and it was much better.

In his first three months of using Byetta he lost about 5 pounds. "The most amazing thing is that after being hungry for most of my life, I can actually say that I now know what it's like for 'normal' people," he says. "I can push the plate away. It does leave me with an interesting dilemma. I used food as a comfort—and now I have to find other ways to be kind to myself. It's the best problem I ever had."

But he wrote me again later. His worst problem was changing his health insurance provider. He lives in Connecticut, and ConnectiCare won't pay for Byetta. Although he was doing wonderfully on it and losing weight, his doctor and health care team have been fighting in vain for it for more than a year. "I have spent the same year on a variety of oral drugs (mostly metformin and sulfonylurea combinations) and nothing has worked as well as Byetta to regulate my blood glucose, not to mention curbing my carbohydrate appetite. You would think they would be happy to pay it in the hope of avoiding complications that will cost them more."

weight control, which is only a happy side effect. Byetta is supposed to be used by people who have "inadequate glycemic control" on metformin, a sulfonylurea, or a thiazolidinedione. In practice, inadequate control generally means an A1C of 7.0 or more. Technically, it is an off-label use to for doctors to prescribe Byetta to people with diabetes whose A1C is better than 7.0. Still, my A1C was 6.8 when my doctor initially prescribed Byetta for me. But there was certainly no question that I needed it for weight loss, even if not for glucose control.

YOU CAN TAKE BYETTA WITH OTHER DRUGS

The original FDA approval of Byetta was only for people taking metformin alone or a sulfonylurea alone or metformin in combination with a sulfonylurea. But in December 2006, the FDA approved its use with the class of drugs known as thiazolidinediones, or TZDs for short. The two available brand-name TZDs are Avandia and Actos. No studies of using Byetta with other drugs for controlling diabetes are finished yet. These other drugs are insulin, D-phenylalanine derivatives like Starlix, meglitinides like Prandin, and alpha-glucosidase inhibitors like Precose or Glyset.

SOME OF YOU CAN'T USE BYETTA

Even more limitations surround the use of Byetta. Women who are pregnant, plan to become pregnant, or who are breast-feeding should talk to their doctor before considering it. One of the most important limitations is that people who have severe kidney disease need to avoid using it. The FDA has also not approved it for children, because Amylin hasn't tested it yet for pediatric use.

When you take medication that needs to be absorbed rapidly, or you depend on reaching a peak concentration, Byetta can get in the way, since it is such a potent inhibitor of gastric emptying. For example, if you are taking a contraceptive, an antibiotic, or Tylenol (acetaminophen), you need to take it at least one hour before the Byetta injection. If you need to take one of these drugs with food, take it with the meal or snack when you don't take Byetta or simply skip that Byetta injection.

FORGET IT IF YOUR STOMACH IS PARALYZED

Another limitation is severe gastrointestinal disease. This includes gastroparesis, which quite a few people with diabetes have—and not everyone who has it knows it. When you take Byetta, your stomach empties slower. That's a good thing, because it helps you lose weight and reduce your blood glucose levels. But a common complication of diabetes called gastroparesis—literally, paralyzed stomach—also causes food to remain in the stomach. That's not a good thing, in part because it can make controlling your blood glucose levels difficult. High blood glucose levels can lead to gastroparesis by causing nerve damage. At the same time, high blood glucose levels make people with type 2 diabetes excellent candidates for Byetta. But if you have gastroparesis and take Byetta, you are supposed to tell your doctor. This assumes, of course, that you know you have gastroparesis. For a condition that few people have ever heard about, gastroparesis is awfully common. Up to 5 million Americans have it.

According to the Wyoming Diabetes Prevention and Control Program, "It is estimated that approximately 25 percent of diabetic patients have gastroparesis, although many patients with gastroparesis remain undiagnosed." Gastroparesis "frequently occurs in people with either type 1 or type 2 diabetes," says the National Center for Chronic Disease Prevention and Health Promotion. "Symptoms of gastroparesis include heartburn, nausea, vomiting of undigested food, an early feeling of fullness when eating, weight loss, abdominal bloating, erratic blood glucose levels, lack of appetite, gastroesophageal reflux, and spasms of the stomach wall."

Not surprisingly, fullness, weight loss, and lack of appetite are the most common side effects of Byetta. It is for these side effects that many people—myself included—take Byetta. Isn't it strange that Byetta's slow stomach emptying works so much better for us than the way gastroparesis does it?

Do You Have the Right Genes for Byetta?

The biggest mystery about Byetta is why some people are so successful at losing a lot of weight on it and others are not. I have heard of some people who have lost very little weight, if any, when they take Byetta. The difference may be in our genes. Some preliminary scientific research indicates that some of us may have a polymorphism or mutation in the receptor for GLP-1, which is the site of action for Byetta. People often use the terms "polymorphism" and "mutation" interchangeably.

But technically a mutation is a rare change in a DNA sequence, while a polymorphism is a common variation.

The key to explaining why some people respond to Byetta and others don't may be in an article in the August 2005 issue of a highly technical journal called *Regulatory Peptides*. These are peptides that regulate physiological processes, including GLP-1. The journal has nothing to do with governmental regulation, as I thought at first. This study reported, "Glucagon-like peptide-1 (GLP-1) and its cognate receptor play an important physiological role in maintaining blood glucose homeostasis. A GLP-1 receptor (GLP-1R) polymorphism . . . has been recently identified in a patient with type 2 diabetes but was not found in non-diabetic control subjects. . . . Sequence variability of the GLP-1R within the human population can result in substantial loss-of-function."

The study's lead author is Martin Beinborn, MD, a pharmacologist and assistant professor at Tufts–New England Medical Center in Boston. He told me that I need to be cautious about not overinterpreting what they discovered, since they found it in just one person who has diabetes. He went on to say, "It sounds somewhat plausible to speculate that the polymorphism was a loss of function, so that endogenous GLP-1 acts less efficiently in this person. And if he were treated with [exogenous] GLP-1 or exendin, he would probably react less than a normal person."

We don't even know how frequent this polymorphism is in the general population, according to Dr. Beinborn. It is a possibility that it might be the answer to the Byetta mystery, but we don't know for sure. Dr. Beinborn tells me that other scientists are now planning to study a large number of people to see if they carry this polymorphism. He says that he brought the study to Amylin's attention. A test for the polymorphism would be technically feasible, "just a simple sequencing thing," he says. But consent of the people tested would be required. "It is still a big question what makes a difference," he says in conclusion. "And polymorphisms like the one we described may be part of the answer. It is probably not as simple as to say that it is in a single receptor; it is in a full spectrum of different receptors that make people more or less susceptible." My guess is that I don't have this polymorphism, because Byetta is working so well for me. I hope that you don't have it either.

CAN YOU EVER STOP BYETTA?

If you have type 2 diabetes and are among those people who can benefit from Byetta, it is likely to help you to lose weight. But once you start Byetta, do you have to take it forever or at some point can you come off it? This is a question that several people have posed to me via e-mail and in person. I have bene-fited so much from Byetta personally that getting off it is the fur-thest thing from my mind. The injections twice a day and the discipline to take them before breakfast and dinner seem a small price to pay for the advantages of weight loss and control that Byetta gives me.

So far, no one has been able to take Byetta for more than two or three years. It first became available in April 2005, although a few people in earlier clinical trials continue to take it. So no one really knows if most of us will have to continue to take it.

Certainly, some people will be able to put their diabetes into re-mission after using Byetta for a while and then stopping it. But my guess is that without Byetta, most of us would revert to our old ways of eating too much because our appetites are too great.

Maybe we won't need Byetta itself. Within a few years we have good reason to think that we will be able to take a long-acting version of Byetta. Already, Byetta's closest cousin, exe-natide LAR, seems to be doing well in clinical trials. If we are lucky, maybe some day we will have to take only one shot a week or one a month to get the same or even better benefits than we now get from taking two shots of Byetta every day.

9

PROBLEMS
WITH BYETTA

The big problem that I had with Byetta was to find a doctor who had heard of it and would prescribe it for me. After that, it was a piece of cake. Good thing, too, because I haven't eaten any cake since then.

YOU DON'T HAVE NEEDLE PHOBIA, DO YOU?

Before Byetta became available, most of the so-called experts thought that its biggest problem would be that it has to be taken by injection. But for almost all users, it's no problem, probably because the injections are much less painful than the finger-sticks that you use to check your blood glucose. Still, more than one person starting out to take Byetta felt like the person who wrote on a Byetta support group. She wrote that she had "weeks of abject fear staring at that pen before I worked up the courage to stick myself with it."

I know what she means, although I am more of a daredevil. Yesterday, as I prepared to take my morning shot of Byetta in my stomach, I reflected on the reluctance I originally had. I know that it was totally irrational, because I had seen my wife shooting up insulin without flinching. I knew; too, that the stomach has almost no nerve endings, so we hardly feel the shot. Any reluctance to do fingerstick tests is a lot more rational. That's one reason why alternative site testing may make sense at some times.

Needle phobia certainly isn't rational. It often starts in childhood, when you receive vaccines and other injections with what look like horse needles. Nowadays, the needles that people with diabetes use for their injections of diabetes drugs are much thinner and shorter. Modern 31 gauge needles are so thin, in fact, that I can't see them without my glasses. They are much shorter too, sometimes just $^3/_{16}$ of an inch long.

It helps to see someone else inject herself or himself, as I watched my wife. It's not like lancing your finger, which often does hurt. I would have been much more reluctant to start testing my blood glucose at first if the pharmacist hadn't showed me by lancing her own finger.

Strangely, as common as needle phobia is, few studies of the condition exist. The professional literature in the government's huge MEDLINE database has just 38 citations. By comparison, I found 214,594 citations for diabetes mellitus. So I guess that it's better to have diabetes than to have needle phobia. At least we know a lot more about it. But if you have both conditions, you've got a problem. Since we don't have a cure yet for diabetes, you need to find a cure for needle phobia.

You Don't Need to Keep It Too Cool

Another problem with Byetta has now disappeared. This was the need to keep it cool but not too cold. Originally, Amylin said that we should protect it from light and store it a refrigerator or use cool gel packs between doses. But if it got frozen, we shouldn't use it. Now, however, Amylin has successfully petitioned the FDA for a label change on refrigeration. Byetta still needs to be kept below 77 degrees F (25 degrees C), away from the light, and never frozen. Now, however, Daniel Bradbury, who was then the company's president and who is now its chief executive officer, says that the company had "demonstrated the stability of Byetta at room temperature for the full 30-day pen lifespan."

You Need to Drink

When you take Byetta, you need to drink. Lots of water. "What's the biggest risk with taking Byetta?" my primary care physician asked me recently. After thinking for a moment, I responded, "It must be the nausea that some people have." He disagreed. "It's dehydration." Actually, nausea and dehydration are linked. Dehydration can be the result of nausea as well as of vomiting and diarrhea. You can also get dehydrated simply by not drinking enough water with the smaller amount of food that you eat when you take Byetta. Of course, you can also get dehydrated if you don't take Byetta. When your diabetes is uncontrolled or untreated, you have a high risk of being dehydrated.

You Can Avoid Nausea Nastiness

For many people, the biggest problem with taking Byetta is the nausea that it often causes, not having to inject it or keep it cool. In the clinical trials, nausea was the most common adverse reaction. Almost half—44 percent—said that they had nausea. Since Byetta is based on naturally occurring GLP-1, which delays gastric emptying, it's not surprising that it makes

---

PROFILE

Ellen Ann (Annie) Myers
Got Dehydrated

"I have a 32-year-old son and a 29-year-old daughter who have never seen me under 300 pounds until recently," Annie Myers says. "My husband and children are so excited to see me at this new weight. It's been more than 30 years since I was below 300, and I have had to replace all my clothes several times. That's a good kind of problem to have! I don't feel proud about the weight loss, because the Byetta did most of the work. The weight just came off."

While she says that "the weight didn't come off very fast," Annie lost 86 pounds in her first 14 months on Byetta. She's down to 216. Before trying Byetta, Annie lost almost 50 pounds with diet and exercise and metformin. It took her almost three years to do that and she says that it was hard work. When her weight stopped coming off, her doctor started her on Byetta.

It was for "the side effect of weight loss" that he switched her to Byetta. At the time, her A1C was quite low, 5.5. Now, it is a low normal 4.8. But problems came up when she started Byetta. The first one was that she quickly *gained* 20 pounds. "I felt the fullness, but

some people nauseous. But the nausea seldom lasts more than a week or so, particularly when we learn to listen to our bodies.

When I started on Byetta, I dreaded the nausea. But I felt a little nauseous for only about three hours after my first injection, and it never returned. I think the reason I had almost no nausea was because I changed what—and how much—I ate at the same time that I started on Byetta. I was so fearful of the nausea demon that I ate very little. In fact, I am still eating very

at the time didn't realize it meant I had eaten enough. All my life I never knew when I was full." She says that other people who use Dr. Bill Quick's Byetta Web site encouraged her, and then she started to do well. Still, she had to face two more problems. Her next problem was constipation, but when her doctor added metformin back, that took care of it. Her last problem was several bouts of dizziness. Testing showed that she was going too low, several episodes of blood glucose levels between 23 and 50. Her doctor suggested that she eat every three hours, and now she rarely goes below 65.

"I didn't have any other side effects and still don't," Annie says. "I never changed my diet on purpose, but I did begin to crave better food like fruits and vegetables. All my old favorites are no longer appealing. Some days I actually have to force myself to eat. I was a binge eater, and now I can't stand those foods that I binged on."

Annie's most recent report is that her doctor took her off Byetta. "He wasn't pleased that I lost 18 pounds in six weeks and found I am very dehydrated. I am off the 10 mcg Byetta pen until further notice, because he said it works too well for me now. He says that he will put me back on the 5 mcg Byetta pen if my blood glucose goes too high."

little, but that is not because of fear of nausea but rather because my appetite is much less now. So I am no expert on nausea. I'm not a doctor either, so I can't give medical advice. But I know a lot of people who use Byetta and know how to dig out information.

It's a shame that some people give up on Byetta because of nausea when they start using it. These are the very people who can benefit the most. Their bodies are telling them that they

EATING STRATEGIES

1. The first eating strategy is small meals and maybe more meals or snacks. When we have heartburn, our body is talking to us. When we have nausea, it's screaming.
2. The second eating strategy is to eat slowly. We are much less likely to eat past the point of satiation when we slow down.
3. What to eat is the third eating strategy. "I have to remember to keep the fat and spices minuscule," one Byetta user wrote. "Definitely avoid spicy or fatty foods," another Byetta user wrote. For example, "I can eat a hamburger, but not a hot dog."
   Minimizing the amount of fat that we eat is key. The problem with fat is that it is "energy dense" and therefore harder to digest. Fat has more than twice as many calories per ounce as protein, sugar, or starch. Because of this, fatty food can fool us into eating too much. We tend to assess our food intake by the size of the portion, which doesn't work when comparing fatty food to the rest of our diet. As a result, we have a weak innate ability to recognize those foods that have a high energy density.
   Instead of energy-dense fats, our bodies are designed for "nutrient-dense" foods. Nutrient-dense foods have a high ratio of nutrients to calories; they are rich in nutrients when compared to their caloric content. While this certainly excludes fatty foods, it also excludes foods high in "empty calories," anything

need a lot less food than they have been eating, so they stand to benefit from the greatest weight loss. While some people find success with either prescription or over-the-counter (OTC) drugs, many more minimize the nausea with different eating strategies. I am in the second camp. My guess is that more people take Byetta to lose weight than to reduce blood glucose. That is certainly my motivation. The weight loss comes naturally and easily from the reduction in hunger. If we listen to our

loaded with sugar or high-fructose corn syrup. These sweeteners don't give us anything but sweetness and calories. Alcohol too gives us nothing but empty calories (and a buzz or more). Nutrient-dense foods are those foods, like fruit and vegetables, that give us substantial amounts of vitamins and minerals and relatively few calories.

4. When to eat is the fourth eating strategy. The general advice for Byetta is to eat from 1 to 60 minutes after taking it. People who have waited more than an hour have reported nausea. In fact, the sooner you eat something after taking Byetta the less the chance of nausea. "If I eat just as soon as I take the injection, it is much better," another Byetta user wrote. "I found that if I inject about 20 minutes before eating, it is the perfect timing for me. I must eat *within* one hour of taking the injection. A word of advice—don't take the Byetta and then forget to eat. I did that this morning. Family crisis. Took the shot and never ate breakfast. I had a miserable day feeling tired and weak. Whatever you do, make sure you eat something, even if it's only a bowl of cereal."

5. The fifth tip is that different foods affect people differently. High-fat foods may be the worst culprits. But whenever you have a bad experience with a particular food, it's best to go easy on it the next time.

bodies, we know when our stomachs are full. But if we keep on eating—the way we always did in the bad old days before Byetta—we are bound to feel the nausea.

YOU CAN AVOID NAUSEA WITH GINGER

Some foods help a lot of people in dealing with nausea. By far the food recommended the most often is ginger in its many forms—including ginger tea, ginger snaps, ginger gum, ginger ale, and ginger pills. One woman wrote that her experience is based less on Byetta and more on pregnancy, "where the nausea can be much worse." She found that natural food stores have one of the best remedies, "ginger ale made with real ginger and no high-fructose corn syrup."

One of my favorite Certified Diabetes Educators wrote me with her ginger tip:

"For a really yummy antinausea concoction, you can make your own fresh ginger root tea. Chop into very small pieces some fresh ginger. (Using a food processor gets it really fine.) If you like lemon, you can add a whole chopped-up lemon, including the peel, to the ginger root. Cover the ginger (and lemon, if you're using it) with water. Heat it to a gentle simmer, and simmer for about an hour or so. Strain out the ginger pieces, and add water (hot or cold) until it's a strength you like. Sweeten it with your sweetener of choice. I use Splenda. My daughter (who doesn't have diabetes) uses honey. I have a friend who uses stevia. What you end up with is ginger ale without the fizz. If you want a fizzy concoction, use club soda to dilute the ginger water."

Others have recommended a cup of hot water sipped slowly, sugar-free mints, chamomile tea, saltines, rice crackers, antacids, Sea-Band Sea Sickness Wristbands, hypnosis, walking, and deep breaths. The wristbands go around your wrists and use acupressure to relieve nausea. You can find them at drugstores. Walgreens calls them "Travel Ease." The recommendation for hypnosis doesn't seem strange to me, considering the power of suggestion. "I wonder if anyone here has tried hypnosis to deal with nausea?" a correspondent wrote me. "I started thinking about this as a result of the Amylin rep telling me that in the Byetta trials that 44 percent of the participants on Byetta reported at least some nausea—and that 18 percent of the participants receiving the placebo had nausea, too."

One person found that taking a long walk helps. It's a good idea in any case! Read all about what walking and hiking can do for your health in a subsequent chapter on "**Aerobic Exercise.**" Another wrote, "I find that if I take a deep breath almost until it hurts and hold my breath for as long as I can and let it out slowly, it generally goes away. If there is no effect the first time, I repeat it."

If none of these strategies work, you might try either an OTC or prescription drug. I think of these as a last resort, because it seems a shame to take a drug to counteract another drug. This can become a vicious circle. I was able to find only two OTC drugs that people recommended for nausea from Byetta. One is Emetrol, which is a mixture of glucose, fructose, and phosphoric acid, and comes in syrup form. This means, of course that it is high glycemic, so it will at least temporarily raise your blood glucose. The other is Prilosec OTC (omeprazole), which most people usually use for frequent heartburn. Prilosec is also available by prescription, which might be a consideration if your health insurance copay is less than the OTC price.

By far, the most commonly recommended prescription drug for nausea is the old standby, Phenergan (promethazine). People on Byetta have also recommended Zofran, metoclopramide (the generic of Reglan), and Prochlorperazine. Like all drugs, they have side effects, some of them serious. There's no point in my going into the pros and cons of these prescription drugs here. Your doctor will decide which one, if any, of these to prescribe.

Bear in mind that Byetta is the synthetic form of Gila monster venom. So you might want to try the half-serious advice that the Diabetes_And_Byetta group offers: "Try to think like a lizard. Avoid what would make a lizard nauseous."

10

WHEN
BYETTA FAILS

The Rev. John L. Dodson is the poster boy for the Byetta revolution. The *New York Times* featured and photographed him in perhaps the most influential article ever about Byetta, which ran on March 2, 2006. That article reported that John had then lost almost 60 pounds since starting Byetta in June 2005. By the end of June 2006, he had lost 88 pounds.

Then, in the middle of August, as John told me later, Byetta stopped working for him to lose more weight. John was sure that his blood glucose would rise, but it didn't. His A1C remained at 6.0 and his twice-daily blood glucose tests ran then between 73 and 110. But John's appetite came roaring back. His weight returned with it. In the next three months he gained back 15 pounds.

"I couldn't stop grazing," John recalls. "One night I ate a whole quart of ice cream." Desperate, John tried everything that he and his endocrinologist, Dr. Joe Prendergast, could think of—hoodia, phentermine, and "even a couple of those preparations 'guaranteed to help you lose weight' that they sell in health stores. I was getting depressed and couldn't believe what was happening," he recalls. "I was less effective and feeling pretty much a failure. There was nothing I did that was successful. I didn't have any willpower in the face of my enemy—my appetite."

He stopped tracking his weight regularly. "I never get on the scales when I'm not losing weight," John told me. "That is an unwritten law when you are gaining. We are great deniers—at least I am." Finally, in October 2006, John says that he decided he "had to do something or die."

"Isn't that a bit extreme?" I asked him. "No, that's how I felt," John replied. "I'm dead if I go back to where I was, and I would not make it. I am still scared to death I am going to lose it all. Constant vigilance!"

JOHN DECIDES TO GET BACK ON TRACK

Eventually, John figured out the way to get back on the weight loss track. Take more Byetta. How did you think of that? I asked him. "It was because of a statement that Dr. Joe made," John told me, "even though I didn't realize the importance of it at the time."

Dr. Joe said that the best way to lose weight is to repeat the method that you were successful with before, John continued. "As I drove back home from my appointment with him, I thought more about what he had said. The only thing that has ever been successful for me was Byetta. So, I should look to Byetta for the answer. And that's when I decided to increase the Byetta dosage to four times a day."

For a week John took two shots of 10 mcg of Byetta in the morning and two more shots at night. It was too much. At the end of the week he got violently ill. So John cut back to three shots a day, sometimes varying it with just the usual two shots. If he doesn't eat lunch, then he takes two shots at night before dinner. "The danger zone for me is eating after dinner," John says. "If I am eating after dinner, I know I am out of control."

By the end of October 2006, John had lost half of the weight he gained back when he was out of control. His weight is now 80 pounds less than when he started to take Byetta on June 13, 2005. "I am clearly on the path of losing weight again," John concludes. "It feels so great! "When I am losing weight, I feel

INSURANCE COVERAGE

Most insurers will cover Byetta through the pharmacy benefit, which is typically managed by a pharmacy benefit manager, or PBM.

Byetta is available by prescription at both retail and mail order pharmacies.

The copayment for which you are responsible varies by insurer.

People who 65 and older and some others are eligible for Medicare. You can find information on the Medicare drug benefit by calling toll-free 800-MEDICARE (800-633-4227) or by visiting www.medicare.gov.

People who do not have adequate insurance or the means to afford Byetta may qualify for the Patient Assistance Program that the manufacturer created. You can obtain the application form online at www.amylin.com/pdf/Byetta_PAP_App.pdf, by calling or 800-330-7647, or by writing:

Amylin Patient Assistance Program
P.O. Box 8435
Gaithersburg, MD 20898

really successful. It makes me happy. I can hardly wait for each day to come, because I know that I am going to lose more weight."

A few years ago John retired as a pastor, but then he started a second career as a fund-raiser for his church. At the end of 2006, he retired for good and lives in Felton, California, near Santa Cruz. John and I have been corresponding since January, when he wrote me about my article "Stalking Byetta." His encouragement for me to start taking Byetta even if I couldn't work out insurance coverage did a lot to get me started on it a few days later.

Since that time, John has been my role model. In mid-October, a consulting contract took me to Santa Cruz, where I used to live, and John graciously invited me to stay at his home for the three days I was there. We had a wonderful time together, swapping stories about Byetta and the rest of our lives, hiking our favorite trail, and eating (small meals) at local restaurants. Then, in January 2007, John stayed with my wife and me in Boulder, Colorado. Through Byetta we have become close friends and learned that we have many other interests in common.

JOHN FINDS SUPPORT FOR SUPPLEMENTAL SHOTS

John decided on his own to increase his Bytta dose. But he gets solid support now from Dr. Joe and another endocrinologist. Dr. Joe says that Amylin Pharmaceuticals, the company that developed Byetta, discouraged him from having his patients go on Byetta three times a day. They said that, based on their data, it wouldn't help. So he temporarily left it there. But now he thinks that trying three times a day might not be unreasonable for people whose weight loss has stalled. So far, John is Dr. Joe's only patient who is taking more than the usual two daily shots of Byetta. "But, emboldened by his success, I will do more," Dr. Joe says. He says that he has also had two or three patients who had weight to lose and were perfect candidates for Byetta. But from the first, it didn't work for them. "At the time I never thought to recommend that they take Byetta three times a day," he told me. "But now I would."

Dr. Alan Rubin, an endocrinologist in San Francisco, also has a patient who successfully experimented with taking more than the standard two daily shots of Byetta. Dr. Rubin is the author of *Diabetes for Dummies*, which two years ago I reviewed in my "Diabetes Update" newsletter. Dr. Rubin also has one of the best diabetes podcasts, which you can hear on his Web site or download to iTunes.

"One of my patients who was on the maximum dose of Byetta was not losing weight and not showing much improvement in blood sugar," Dr. Rubin says on his Byetta Healthcast #44 of September 25, 2006. "On his own he increased his maximum nighttime dose above the 10 mcg. He immediately began to lose weight. His blood sugar levels have become normal. He looks and feels much better than before. His hemoglobin A1C has fallen into the normal range."

Based on that experience, Dr. Rubin says, he had another patient take two shots of Byetta before dinner. She, too, is now doing much better, he says. Consequently, Dr. Rubin discussed this approach with a scientist at Eli Lilly, which markets

Byetta together with Amylin. "Although they recommend a maximum of 10 mcg twice daily," Dr. Rubin concludes, "they, too, found that as the dose is raised, there is more weight loss. As a result of this I plan to increase the dose of Byetta in my patients who fail to lose much weight. As long as they can afford the cost of the medication, I will offer it to them."

Anyone taking Byetta more than twice a day needs to be prepared to pay for it. I doubt if many health insurance plans will cover it—and Byetta is expensive. John has been on Byetta a lot longer than I have used it. I am already thinking ahead that I may have to go to Byetta three times daily, in part because of research that Dr. Joe reported in his newsletter, "Weight, Weight Don't Tell Me!" He reports, "All diets seem to work for about 12 months, but seem to cease working at the end of the 12 months." Byetta is, of course, not a diet. It's much more than that. And so far, I am still losing weight and have been for more than a year. My blood glucose, blood pressure, and cholesterol levels are down, while my energy level is way up. But I'm ready to change to three shots a day, and pay whatever it costs, if I need to in order to control my weight. Like John, I know that getting and keeping this weight off is a matter of life or death.

THE GLP-1
LIFESTYLE

When is a diet not a diet? When it's the way that you want to eat. When it's not feeling that you are depriving yourself. When it's not just a question of willpower. In those senses, there really isn't any such thing as a GLP-1 or Byetta diet. Byetta is, of course, the first drug based on glucagonlike peptide-1 or GLP-1. But many more are coming, so I sometimes call this the GLP-1 diet, although it's really a lifestyle, not a diet. Confusing enough? Certainly. But terminology is one thing. The reality of what and how much we eat when we use a GLP-1 drug couldn't be simpler.

IT CAN END YOUR HUNGER

The key point is that this lifestyle—or eating plan or just plain following the principles of good nutrition—when we use Byetta or one of the forthcoming GLP-1s—couldn't be more different from anything the world has ever known before. The reason for this is that GLP-1 suppresses the appetite. Several other ways to say this all make the same point: You aren't hungry all the time. You feel full on a lot less food. Scientists know this as satiety. After all, the GLP-1 that Byetta mimics is a synthetic version of what the Gila monster uses. The Gila monster needs to suppress its appetite a lot more than we do. Unlike us, it eats only a few times a year.

Byetta makes eating less and losing weight possible. It doesn't cause weight loss without changing the diet. It is not automatic. That's why people in the clinical trials for Byetta lost so few pounds compared with people who consciously are trying to lose weight. "Patients were not required to follow any specified diet or exercise plan," say Amylin Pharmaceuticals and Eli Lilly on the Byetta Web site.

Now that I am on Byetta, I feel full almost all the time, so I almost always eat very little. When I do eat a normal-sized meal, as I have two or three times when I went out to dinner, I paid the price with a few hours of heartburn afterward.

Do You Need Willpower?

Willpower is the *internal strength* of will to carry out our decisions, wishes, or plans. Do we need a lot of willpower to lose weight on Byetta or one of the other GLP-1 mimetics that almost certainly will be here by 2009? Before GLP-1 mimetics became available, dieting certainly required a lot of willpower. And it rarely worked, as Gina Kolata forcefully points out in her new book *Rethinking Thin*. She tracked a group of volunteers in an intensive two-year program at the University of Pennsylvania. They invariably gained back the weight they lost. But using a GLP-1 mimetic isn't dieting, and now willpower is no longer such a big thing. The big difference is that these new drugs give us *external strength* to fight off the urge to gorge.

The proof of this is that people in the clinical trials of Byetta who did as they were told did lose weight. The people who ran the trials told these volunteers not to change what they were doing—specifically not to change their diet or exercise habits. That's probably why so many people in the clinical trials experienced nausea. Nonetheless, the volunteers still lost weight. Typically, however, they didn't lose a lot of weight.

The GLP-1 mimetics work with us to help us lose weight. Since they make our stomachs empty more slowly, we feel full longer. Since they also signal our hypothalamus, they tell our heads that we have eaten enough. The trick for us in working with these drugs is simply to listen to what our bodies are telling us. That's not so much willpower as it is awareness.

The role of willpower in weight loss is less in what we eat than in the exercise we do. It does take willpower to start exercising after years of surviving without it. Exercise not only burns calories, it speeds up our metabolism. There's more about this in the chapter "Metabolism and Exercise." Starting to exercise is a major change in our habits.

YOU MAY NEED SUPPLEMENTAL NUTRITION

Since I eat so little, I know that I have to be especially careful to get all the vitamins and minerals that my body needs. This is the same problem that people following the Calorie Restriction (CR) diet have in spades. Followers of that diet, popularized by

Roy Walford and his daughter Lisa in various books, call it a lifestyle or way of eating, rather than a diet. Actually, it is more of a way of not eating. No diet restricts what you can eat more severely. People follow the CR lifestyle in hopes that they can delay aging so that they can increase their lifespan.

Some people call this a starvation diet. One article says that with it you can "Diet your way to a long, miserable life!" My guess is that most people who have started on the CR did find it miserable and gave up. But some good scientific evidence for it exists, and I can't fault it—as long as you don't feel miserable on it. Besides feeling hungry almost all the time, people who do CR have to make sure that they get as much good nutrition as

PROFILE
ANN WILLIAMS FINDS WILLPOWER

Ann Williams is one of my favorite Certified Diabetes Educators, one who has helped me in my writing about diabetes for years. She also has diabetes and also takes Byetta.

Before Byetta, willpower was never enough for her. Ann says that before she used Byetta, "no matter how hard she tried, weight loss just did not follow effort." Now the effort pays off for her, especially if she pays attention to when she feels full and applies effort intelligently—to increasing her exercise. "I find physical activity plus Byetta actually decreases appetite for me, making the portion control effort more sustainable. I, and most other people, do need physical activity for sustainable weight loss," Ann says.

On Byetta, her diet has also changed. "I have much less taste for meat and am eating tiny portions, if any at all. That alone accounts for some of my weight loss."

they can with the small amount of food that they eat. For that reason, the Walfords originally called it the Calorie Restriction with Optimal Nutrition (CRON) diet. The best way to get optimal nutrition is to avoid junk food and empty calories.

This means, first of all, to avoid products that have sugar or high-fructose corn syrup in them. But more than simply avoiding bad foods, they have to reach out to good ones. I discuss the best and worst foods in subsequent chapters of this book.

Second, it's probably wise to supplement the good food you eat with a multivitamin and especially the B vitamins that help defend your body against high levels of **homocysteine**. This risk factor for heart disease is especially important for people with diabetes, which is linked to high levels of it.

Most of us with diabetes also need more magnesium and vitamin D than we are getting in our diet. I supplement my diet with 300 mg of magnesium citrate daily. I also have drastically increased how much vitamin D I take on the basis of a new analysis.

Some people take far more supplements than I do. I'm sure that some of these help them. But for most, if not all, of these supplements, scientific proof is scant, if not lacking altogether. Whenever I hear recommendations that we take one of these supplements, I make sure to check out the evidence. Steven Bratman, a medical doctor practicing in Colorado, developed an encyclopedic resource that he calls the "Natural Health Encyclopedia," formerly "The Natural Pharmacist." You can find it on some Web sites as "The Natural Pharmacist" or "The Complementary Therapies Natural Health Encyclopedia."

Many public libraries offer it as the "Natural and Alternative Treatments" database.

Because of Byetta, I take a few more supplements than I did before and have radically changed my diet. It is lower in calories, lower in **carbohydrates**, and lower glycemic. While "lower caloric" and "lower carbohydrate" are concepts that we all understand, what I mean by "lower glycemic" might need a bit of explaining. For that, please see the next chapter. What Byetta has done for me—in addition to helping me reduce my blood glucose levels, which in itself is no little thing—is to keep me from *thinking* about food all the time. This has made it so much easier to choose only healthy food to eat. Eating healthier has made me feel so much better. I can now control the food I eat instead of having the food I eat control me. It is freeing.

Make Sure You Eat Enough

Maybe the strangest problem when we take Byetta or one of the forthcoming GLP-1 mimetics is to eat enough. It's not just vitamins and minerals and supplements that we need. We have to get enough calories and protein, too. It is a balance. For years, most of us have been getting too many calories and too much protein, but now, with the help of a drug that can dramatically reduce our appetite, we have to be careful not to go too far in the other direction. We can actually set our sights too high and try too hard to lose weight. I know that sometimes I did. If you don't eat enough each day, you can drive your body into starvation mode, where it works all too efficiently to get every bit of nutrition out of the few calories that you give it. Just as we can be too efficient in doing all that we have to do with little physical effort, our bodies can be too efficient for us to lose weight.

When it comes to counting calories, how little is too little? Most people agree that men need at least 1,200 calories per day and women need at least 1,000 calories per day. Skipping breakfast or lunch doesn't help at all to lose weight. In fact, I sometimes try to have not only three meals a day—small ones, to be sure—but also very small snacks in between. That works better to help us lose weight than starving ourselves. Isn't that strange?

Now that I eat so little, making sure that I satisfy my daily protein requirement has been as big a concern for me as counting calories. Most people with diabetes think a lot more about the calories and the carbohydrates and the fat we eat than the amount of protein. Indeed, the typical American diet—which is heavy on calories and especially heavy on meat—provides two or three times as much protein as most of us need. This extra protein not only can prevent weight loss but can even add extra stress on our kidneys and increase our risk of osteoporosis. But when so little food satisfies us, we have to watch carefully how much protein we get. The best resource for determining our daily protein requirement comes from the Food and Nutrition Board of the Institute of Medicine, which is an independent nongovernmental entity that is nonetheless responsible for the recommended dietary allowances of nutrients in the American diet. It says that adult men need 56 grams of good-quality protein per day and that most adult women need 46 grams. Pregnant women and nursing mothers need 71 grams. This means we can get enough protein if we set our minds to it. For example, 4 ounces of chinook salmon or cooked turkey breast gives us 23 grams of top-quality protein. And that is with less than 100 calories. A can of low-sodium, skinless, and boneless sardines in water gives us about 20 grams of protein and about 130 calories. Each of those choices is a great basis for one good meal on the GLP-1 lifestyle.

THE GLYCEMIC AND
SATIETY INDEXES

The glycemic index ranks foods on how they affect our blood glucose levels. This index measures how much your blood glucose increases after you eat. The satiety index ranks foods according to how well they satisfy our hunger. The two concepts have a lot in common. But, strangely, those foods that are low glycemic—those foods that don't spike our blood glucose levels—aren't necessarily those that are low in satiety.

YOUR GLYCEMIC GOODIES

Fatty foods don't satisfy. But they are low glycemic, because only sugars and starches have an immediate effect on blood glucose levels. Boiled potatoes, which are high in starch, do satisfy. So we need to understand both concepts to control our blood glucose without being so hungry that it's hard to lose weight. When you make use of the glycemic index to prepare healthy meals, it helps to keep your blood glucose levels under control. This is especially important for people with diabetes, although anyone who is overweight also stands to benefit from knowing about this relatively new concept in good nutrition.

You can benefit from eating low glycemic in so many ways. When you reduce the glycemic values of the carbohydrates you eat, you improve both the rate of your fat loss and your cardiovascular risk factors. When you eat low glycemic, you get a higher metabolic rate, reduced blood glucose levels after meals, less secretion of insulin, and higher fat oxidation.

When you begin a diet, your metabolic rate usually drops in response to our reduced caloric intake. One recent study found, however, that the metabolic rate drops less on a low-glycemic diet than on a high-carbohydrate diet. This is probably because a low-glycemic diet reduces the amount of muscle loss but doesn't reduce the amount of fat that you lose. Since your muscles burn a lot more calories than fat does, your metabolism stays revved up. A subsequent chapter discusses the crucial importance of metabolism to our continuing weight loss. Studies of large numbers of people with diabetes show that those who keep their blood glucose under tight control are best able to avoid complications. The experts agree that what works best for people with diabetes—and probably for everyone—is regular exercise, very little saturated and no trans fat, less salt, and a high-**fiber** diet. That is excellent advice—as far as it goes.

The real problem is carbohydrates. That's what the glycemic index is all about. Foods high in fat or protein don't cause any immediate rise in your blood glucose level. The conventional wisdom remains that a high-carbohydrate diet is best for people with diabetes. However, some experts recommend a low-carbohydrate diet, because carbohydrates break down

quickly during digestion and can raise blood glucose to danger-
ous levels. A low-glycemic diet avoids both extremes. Many carbohydrate-rich foods have high glycemic values and certainly
are not good in any substantial quantity for people with diabetes, especially anyone who has some weight to lose. Other
carbohydrates break down more slowly, releasing glucose gradually into our bloodstreams. They have lower glycemic values.

The really shocking results of the glycemic index studies are
which foods produce the highest glycemic response. They include many of the starchy foods we eat a lot of, including most
bread, most breakfast cereals, and most potatoes. But table
sugar, technically known as sucrose and long believed to be the
worst thing for people with diabetes, won't raise blood glucose
levels as much and as fast as those starchy foods. Before the development of the glycemic index, beginning in 1981, scientists
assumed that our bodies absorbed and digested simple sugars
quickly, producing rapid increases in our blood glucose level.
This was the basis of the advice to avoid sugar, a proscription recently relaxed by the American Diabetes Association and others.

A more pleasant surprise is the very low glycemic value of a
tasty bean called chana dal, which is the mainstay of the traditional diet of India. Another pleasant surprise is barley, which
has the lowest glycemic value of any grain. Other foods that are
high in carbohydrates but low glycemic include leafy vegetables, beans, pasta, and oats. Acidic fruits also have low glycemic
values. Likewise, vinegar and lemon juice—as in salad dressing—help reduce the glycemic value of a meal.

The glycemic values of foods should not be your only criterion
when selecting what to eat. The total amount of carbohydrate,

the amount and type of fat, and the fiber and salt content are also important dietary considerations. The glycemic index comes into play when you decide which high-carbohydrate foods to eat. But don't let the glycemic index lull you into eating more carbohydrates than your body can handle. The number of grams of carbohydrate you consume is awfully important, too. Make sure that you know the carbohydrate content of the foods you eat by studying the nutritional information on the package.

PROFILE

TimSlim Adds Low-Glycemic Emphasis

Tim Feathers used to call himself Fat Tim. He's now TimSlim, reflecting his weight loss. When he started taking Byetta in July 2005, Fat Tim weighed 293 pounds. Now TimSlim weighs 215.

"Formerly gluttonous and slothful, but now in recovery," Tim-Slim, who is 43, says that he is not only down 78 pounds but also down from a 46-inch waist to one that is 33 to 34 inches. His body fat is also down from 44 percent to 16 percent. His A1C dropped from 8.7 to 5.6. He's also mostly dropped two other diabetes medications he was taking—insulin and Actos. Only when he overloads on carbohydrates does he cover it with a shot of insulin.

Along with Byetta, exercise is a big part of TimSlim's success. He has been a black belt in the martial arts for the last 20 years but says that he lacked dietary discipline until he started Byetta. The biggest change came when he started doing light **resistance training** for about three hours two days a week. He jogs for about an hour a day the other five days of the week. Even Byetta, he says, is no substitute for hard work. "But, it can be done with extreme

Factors such as variety, cooking, and processing may affect a food's glycemic value. Foods particularly sensitive to these factors include bananas, rice, and potatoes. In addition, the glucose response to a particular food may be somewhat individual. So it is probably a good idea to carefully watch your own blood glucose after eating foods you have questions about and determine if they have high or low glycemic value for you. If you find that a specific food produces an unexpected result, either high or low, take note of it and incorporate that knowledge into

diligence. If you can't use your lower body for exercise, then get some dumbbells."

While TimSlim was always heavily into exercise, his new emphasis on nutrition has been quite a change for him, he says. He now eats mostly lean protein—oriented meals with some low-glycemic carbs. He also consumes salmon at least three times a week, takes in flaxseed oil every morning, and uses olive oil almost daily. As long as he is responsible with his diet, Byetta causes no noticeable side effects other than occasional mild nausea and fatigue one and a half hours after injection. In fact, after TimSlim normalized his weight, he found he had a lot more energy. "I think that Byetta literally saved my life."

TimSlim says that he knows now that his weight is totally under his control. So he is going to lose another 20 pounds. "The weight loss keeps going so long as I suppress the desire for 'comfort' eating at night."

His advice for other people with diabetes is to "stick with low-glycemic meals, follow a responsible diet regimen, drink up to eight glasses of clear sugarless fluid daily, *and* be sure to exercise at least 30 minutes daily. Give it six months or so on Byetta while following the advice above. This is a long-term chronic disease that requires a lifetime lifestyle change of diet and exercise."

your meal planning. Also note that the glycemic values of individual foods can vary from study to study. This may be due to variations in the individuals in a particular study, other foods consumed at the same time, or different methods of preparation, since your body can absorb some foods better when they are well cooked.

Most of the foods tested are high in carbohydrates. Some of you may wonder at the gaps—why other high-carbohydrate but low-calorie foods like celery (or tomatoes or similar foods) have never been tested. The problem is a technical one for the testers, because they would be so hard put to get anyone to volunteer to eat 50 grams of carbohydrate from celery—it's just too much celery to think about. This means that you are exceedingly unlikely to eat enough of these foods for them to have much of an influence on your blood glucose level. Essentially, from a glycemic value standpoint, celery and foods like it can be considered free foods.

Some of you may wonder if the glycemic index can predict the effect of a mixed meal containing foods with different values. Studies have shown that it does that job very well, too. You can quite readily predict the glycemic value of a mixed meal. Simply multiply the percent of total carbohydrate of each of the foods by its glycemic value and add up the results to get the glycemic value of the meal as a whole.

Scientists have so far measured the glycemic values of more than 750 high-carbohydrate foods. The key is to eat little of those foods with a high glycemic value and more of those foods with a low value. Low-glycemic foods have a value of 55 or below. But your diet as a whole needs to have an average value of less than 45 so that you can minimize your risk of heart disease.

YOUR SATIETY STUFF

The satiety index is a concept similar to that of the glycemic index. In fact, researchers in the top glycemic index laboratory developed it. The satiety index ranks different foods on their ability to satisfy hunger. Dr. Susanna Holt found that some foods, like croissants, are only half as satisfying as the baseline, white bread. On the other hand, boiled potatoes are more than three times as satisfying, easily the most satisfying food tested. But potatoes in a different form—french fries—did not score well.

"Roughly speaking, the more fiber, protein, and water a food contains, the longer it will satisfy," Dr. Holt told me. "But you have to look at each foodstuff individually—and that is why we think our index will be so useful."

As a group, fruits ranked at the top, with a satiety index 1.7 times more satisfying, on average, than white bread. Carbohydrate-rich foods and protein-rich foods deter nibbling almost as well. Dr. Holt warns, however, that she found big differences between the satisfaction values of individual foods within the same group. Another thing that makes a food satisfying is its sheer bulk. That's probably why lettuce and other salad greens make us feel full without eating many calories.

"Fatty foods are not satisfying, even though people expected them to be," Dr. Holt added. "We think the reason is that fat is seen by the body as a fuel which should be used only in emergencies—it stores it in the cells instead of breaking it down for immediate use. Because it doesn't recognize the fat as energy for immediate use, the body does not tell the brain to cut hunger signals, so we go on wanting more. Carbohydrates are the opposite—they raise blood glucose so the body knows it has gotten enough fuel."

This is just the barest introduction to the fascinating concepts of the glycemic index and the satiety index. Besides Dr. Holt's articles in professional journals and my analysis in *Diabetes Interview* magazine (reprinted on my Web site), little information on the satiety index is yet available. But there's almost too much to read now about the glycemic index. By far, the best books about it are four that Prof. Jennie Brand-Miller wrote with other coauthors and that Marlowe & Company publishes. The basic book is *The New Glucose Revolution*, third edition, 2007. *The Low GI Diet Revolution*, 2005, is the practical companion volume. The third book, *The New Glucose Revolution for Diabetes*, is the most recent, and it specifically applies the concept of the glycemic index to managing diabetes and prediabetes. The fourth book, *The New Glucose Revolution: What Makes My Blood Glucose Go Up . . . and Down?*, gets a special recommendation from me here, because I am one of the coauthors. The second edition of this book came out in 2006. Each of these books includes tables of all the glycemic values.

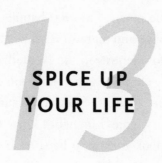

SPICE UP
YOUR LIFE

Some foods that we love to eat are also good for us. My wife claimed that I eat all sorts of bad-tasting things to control my diabetes. But it turns out now that some of the great-tasting things that I love are also healthy. To live a good life with diabetes has to mean, first, that we control our blood glucose. But it also means enjoying the good things in life. I have had diabetes long enough to take for granted that I have to control it every day. At the same time, I know that I have to make each day as good a day as it can be.

REWARDING OURSELVES

For me, living the good life with diabetes starts with enjoying the exercise that I know I need. Everyone likes to do different things, but the exercise that I like to do most is to walk or hike. It takes me to beautiful places where I can be doing something for myself. In the morning, I often promise to reward myself by stopping at my favorite coffee shop for a triple espresso. And I think that it is as important to keep the promises that we make to ourselves as those that we make to other people. Plus, espresso makes me happy. I'm even happier now to read that the caffeine in coffee and espresso has a positive "metabolic effect," according to scientists in the Netherlands who reported on the "Metabolic effects of spices, teas, and caffeine."

These effects are "greater thermogenesis and in some cases . . . greater satiety," they write. I thought I knew what thermogenesis means, but I looked it up to be sure. It means producing heat. One clear sign that what you are eating or drinking that thermogenesis is working for you is when you break out in a sweat from a spicy meal. Sweating is a good thing. It helps us to lose weight. But unless the coffee or espresso is awfully hot, it won't make you sweat. It does contribute to satiety, the sense of feeling full. The authors say that capsaicin, black pepper, ginger, and mixed spices are some good examples of thermogenic foods. Capsaicin is the active component of chili peppers.

PROFILE

JEAN BIANCHI FOUND THAT FOOD TASTES DIFFERENT

When she had been using Byetta for ten months, Jean Bianchi wrote me that food she used to love no longer tastes good to her. She wondered if that was due to the Byetta. It may well have been. But seven months later she told me that the taste of food is now back to normal.

Her blood glucose is also normal now, and she has lost about 10 pounds. "I feel good," she says. "For a 79-year-old woman, I think I am doing really well."

These wonderful plants sure do make us sweat, particularly the habaneros, which are rated at 300,000 Scoville units and above. The spices that I buy are hardly that hot. I generally get my spices from Penzeys Spices, because they are the freshest and are available in the greatest variety. For example, Penzeys offers eight kinds of cinnamon.

COFFEE, TEA, AND YOU

While I often kick off my day drinking espresso at a nearby Internet café, I usually start each morning with a cup of wonderful black coffee from Peet's. The Dutch certainly know a thing or two about coffee. Alfred Peet, who founded my favorite coffee brewing company, came originally from the Netherlands.

The Dutch authors of the new research on the metabolic effects of caffeine also recommend green and black tea. These teas are something that I could well have included above as contributing to living the good life. I drink only the highest-quality teas I can get. For the past decade, I have found them at Upton Tea Imports. I especially love those teas that I can drink straight (without milk, sugar, or lemon). My preferences range widely from the most delicate white teas, which have the least processing of any tea, to lapsang souchong, a black tea that gets its intensely smoky flavor from drying the leaves over a smoldering pine fire. These teas help me get through the afternoons without heavy snacking. Like espresso and coffee, they have great taste without calories. When we combine these drinks with tasty meals that don't add many calories, we get a winning weight loss combination that we can enjoy at the same time.

14

DAVID'S
DIABETES DIET

My food choices are easy. What I eat must do two things for me:

1. Everything must taste great.
2. It must provide great nutrition.

Great taste is subjective and certainly varies from person to person. But great nutrition is objective, even if none of us has all the answers yet. All of us are still learning about nutrition. That's one of the things that makes it especially interesting to study. But we do know the foods that are good for us and those that we should avoid.

So, then, why is diet the most controversial part of controlling diabetes? This controversy rages over just one issue—whether we should be eating a low- or high-carb diet. The most appropriate level of carbohydrates is the only controversial part of the American Diabetes Association's new nutrition recommendations. Some people think that it's too high carb. But my diet is a moderate one, and you can tweak it to include the amount of carbohydrates that you decide is best for you.

What I eat keeps evolving. In the dozen or so years since a doctor diagnosed my diabetes, my diet has changed dozens of times. Nutrition has become one of my biggest interests, and I used to think about what to eat more than I think about sex. Not many men can say that! Judging from the questions I get from my correspondents, women think about diet a lot more than men do. Maybe it's because they have less testosterone. But I guess, instead, that this is because they generally shop and cook for their families. Several recent questions from my correspondents, in fact, prompted me to write about my diet recommendations. For example, Kelly would like to retrain her husband, her son, and herself to eat better. Mary Lee wants to know the easiest eating plan to follow. Kabir wonders if I could make a list of foods that boost our health, are low glycemic, and are full of antioxidants.

OUR BEST FOODS

I don't even have to make a list of the best foods. George Mateljan, the founder and original owner of Health Valley Foods, has thought about food even more than I have. He has a superb list of the world's healthiest foods. If you have Internet access, it's easy to find at www.whfoods.org. I generally agree with George's food choices. The only difference is that I am more concerned with the glycemic values of foods than he is, because I write specifically for people with diabetes.

My pantry is pretty bare compared to most people's. I like to keep it as simple as possible. I keep my recipes simple, too. More than six ingredients—excluding two or three spices—are usually too many for me. My diet would make Linus in the *Peanuts* comic strip happy. He decided not to drink something when he saw what it said on the side of the package. "It's full of ingredients!" he exclaimed.

FRUITS, VEGETABLES, AND LEGUMES

My diet includes almost all the fruits and vegetables. Generally, I prefer to steam the vegetables that I cook, although the microwave is great for winter squash, and boiling is best for cooked greens, like spinach and chard. I go easy on some of those so-called root vegetables—the ones that grow underground—especially potatoes and beets, since they are higher glycemic. For the same reason, I also go easy on dried fruit, like raisins, dates, and prunes. They are certainly great in low doses, but eating a lot of them spikes my blood glucose. Going easy on starches, especially rice, potatoes, and wheat flour, has finally become easy for me. I can do without rice completely (except when I eat out at a Thai restaurant), but I do love potatoes, which also have a lot of nutrition going for them. I have switched from the highest-glycemic potatoes— baked Burbank russets and mashed potatoes—to lower-glycemic varieties—especially fingerlings and small new potatoes—and enjoy them steamed, boiled, or cold in a salad. Legumes are also a wonder food. Chana dal, garbanzo beans, kidney beans, soybeans, and lentils are low glycemic and high in protein.

NUTS AND SEEDS

Nuts and seeds are also important in my diet. Almonds, walnuts, Brazil nuts, and hazelnuts are especially nutritious. Flax seeds, sesame seeds, and pumpkin seeds also offer a lot of the nutrients that we need. Brazil nuts are the best source of selenium, so good, in fact, that the "UC Berkeley Wellness Letter," to which I subscribe, recommends eating no more than five of them a day. Walnuts and flaxseeds are a good source of the essential omega-3 fatty acids. Pumpkin seeds are high in zinc. And I remember to choose unsalted nuts when I shop.

SALAD

One of my favorite lunches or dinners is a salad of vegetables and beans. A large study in the September 2006 issue of the *Journal of the American Dietetic Association* reported that people who eat salads have higher levels of vitamins C and E, folic acid, and carotenoids.

GRAINS, ESPECIALLY BARLEY

Besides fruits, vegetables, and legumes, the other cornerstone of my diet is whole grains. But I seldom eat any grains other than barley, rye, and corn. The other grains, especially most varieties of rice and anything made from wheat flour—including almost all wheat bread, crackers, cookies, and other pastries—are too high glycemic for me. Better bread and cracker choices are pumpernickel—a type of German sourdough bread made with a combination of rye flour and rye meal—and crisp breads made from rye. These are much lower glycemic than bread and crackers made from wheat flour.

Pearl barley has by far the lowest glycemic value of any grain ever tested. Its glycemic value is 25. Next lowest is rye, but only in the form of its whole kernels, with a glycemic value of 34. Corn's glycemic value is quite a bit higher, 53. But pearl barley is not a whole grain, according to the National Barley Foods Council. When processors prepare pearl barley, they strip off most of the bran layer and germ. This removes some of the insoluble fiber, trace minerals, and micronutrients. The government's latest dietary guidelines encourage us to eat whole grains. Its definition of a whole grain is one that "must retain nearly the same relative proportions of bran, germ, and endosperm as the original grain."

The whole-grain form of barley is available, though you may have to search for it at natural food stores or mail order it. It almost certainly has an even lower glycemic value than pearl barley. Whole-grain barley goes by many names, the most common being "hulless barley." I prefer to call it "naked barley." Anyway, that's what processors often call it. So, ironically, naked barley is less processed than pearl barley. It's not what most people have in mind when they put a "Get Naked" bumper sticker on their cars, but it's probably a better idea.

You can get naked barley, aka hulless barley, at a great Internet and mail order source of hulless barley that I have used for years. It's Bob's Red Mill Natural Foods in Milwaukie, Oregon.

This company calls it "whole hull-less barley." It has a similar beige color to that of pearl barley, but it has a pleasant chewy texture and more fiber and nutritional value. Unlike most grains, it takes 4 cups of water to every cup of barley. I learned that lesson the hard way, when I used just a 2 to 1 proportion and produced something that was almost inedible. Nowadays, I cook naked barley in a small rice cooker that I don't use for anything else. Besides eating the barley as a hot cereal, I add it to soups, stews, chili beans, and curries. You can use naked barley everywhere that you formerly used rice.

Naked barley makes a great breakfast with a quite low glycemic value. In fact, I like it so much and it's so little known and yet so good for us that here is the only recipe in this book:

Better Barley Breakfast

$1/4$ cup naked barley and 1 cup water in a small rice
   cooker for as long as it takes (about 40 minutes)

A little cinnamon

A few sliced or slivered almonds

A little nonnutrient sweetener (stevia or Splenda)

A little salt substitute (Sunny Paris or Mural of Flavor
   from Penzeys or Spike)

One tablespoon of freshly ground golden flax seeds

A few fresh blueberries, blackberries, raspberries, or strawberries (washed just before adding them to the bowl)

$2/3$ cup plain unsweetened soy or almond milk (heated in
   microwave for 1 $1/2$ minutes)

I think of this breakfast as real comfort food that happens to be very healthful. It's my usual, but for variety and when I am in a hurry I sometimes prepare a bowl of Whole Control's Golden Barley Cereal, a special, all-natural variety of naked barley flakes. In the United States, we use barley most often as food for our animals and as malt for the beer industry. We have a new demand for it for in ethanol production. But I prefer to eat it naked.

OUR GOOD FATS

At the time of my diabetes diagnosis the conventional wisdom was still that all fats were bad. Nobody woke me and the rest of the world up to the fact that some fats are good fats as much as Udo Erasmus did with his book *Fats That Heal, Fats That Kill*. In addition to the essential omega-3 fats, the good fats are other polyunsaturated ones and those that are monounsaturated. For cooking, the only oil I use is olive oil, which is high in monounsaturated fatty acids. I also eat avocados, which are also among the highest in this good fat.

I am not a vegetarian. For dinner I eat wild fatty fish—particularly salmon—about twice a week during its short season. Otherwise, I supplement my diet with a daily tablespoon of Carlson brand fish oil, which is free of detectable levels of contaminants. The other top choices for omega-3 fatty acids are canned sardines, salmon, and herring. I especially like the Season and Reese brands of sardines that have no added salt, no oil, no skin, and no bones. Omega-3 fatty acids are polyunsaturated fats. But all of the excellent sources that I have been able to find also have some saturated fat. Is that a reason for you to take a pass on them? I think not, because of the benefits that omega-3 provides. Better to cut out all the other sources of saturated fats from your diet.

I also eat bison, both ground and as stew meat. Bison is much lower in saturated fat than beef. And sometimes I cook a boneless, skinless chicken breast, which is also low in saturated fat. I cook salmon, ground bison, and chicken at low temperature in my oven on a cedar roasting plank. This is an easy, simple, and tasty way to prepare these great foods.

FIBER

Because I eat so little now that I am using Byetta, I make sure to get enough fiber. It's generally better to get nutrients from our food rather than from supplements, but few of us, myself included, can readily get enough fiber that way. So with each meal I take four psyllium husk caps. Except for some vegans, almost no one of us gets enough fiber in our diet. On average, American women get 12 grams per day; American men get 18. The experts say that we should get from 25 to 40 grams per day. But when we start taking fiber seriously, we have to take it slowly. If you increase your fiber load too rapidly, it will likely cause intestinal distress.

If anything is a "free food," fiber is. A free food is one that is essentially free of any serious impact on your blood glucose. While in the United States we consider fiber to be a carbohydrate, it won't raise our blood glucose. In Europe, in fact, they don't even count it as a carbohydrate, which can confuse us when we study the nutrition labels on products produced and labeled in a European country.

Fiber actually helps us to control blood glucose spikes. It doesn't have any calories nor any available carbohydrate that can be digested. Some people refer to available carbohydrate as "glycemic," "usable," "net," or "nutritive" carbohydrate. But all of these terms refer to the same thing.

Except for fiber supplements, nothing that we eat is all fiber. Even oat bran has some protein, fat, and available carbohydrate. All plants that we eat for food—including fruits, vegetables, grains, and beans—have some fiber. The key word here is plants. No meat, poultry, seafood, dairy products, eggs, or fats have any fiber.

We can categorize fiber in several ways. The most common way is by type—how easily it dissolves in water. Soluble fiber partially dissolves in water. Insoluble fiber does not dissolve in water. Dietary fiber is the name for these two types together. We need a balance of soluble and insoluble fiber, and both soluble and insoluble fiber fill us up without adding calories. But soluble fiber, in particular, has several major benefits for people with diabetes. By delaying stomach emptying, it slows the digestion of starches and sugars and thereby reduces blood glucose spikes. It also decreases the level of cholesterol in our blood, which reduces our risk of heart disease, the main complication of diabetes. Insoluble fiber, when taken with enough water, promotes bowel regularity and may help prevent hemorrhoids, spastic colon, diverticulitis, and colon cancer. However, it doesn't lower cholesterol.

Oatmeal and oat bran have received most of the good publicity about their fiber. That's because about half of their fiber is soluble. And that's why the FDA has allowed a health claim on oat products. Recently, the FDA allowed that claim on barley products too, because half of its fiber also is soluble. But some other foods have even more soluble stuff in a serving. Beans are the winners here. Brussels sprouts and citrus are also highly soluble.

The best sources of insoluble fiber include whole grains, nuts and seeds, and vegetables such as green beans, cauliflower, zucchini, and celery. The first ingredient in Kellogg's popular breakfast cereal All-Bran (including its All-Bran Bran Buds, All-Bran Original, and All-Bran Extra Fiber) is wheat bran, which is four-fifths insoluble fiber. However, All-Bran also includes high-fructose corn syrup, which is probably worse for us than sugar (see the "Sugar" chapter).

Another way to categorize fiber is by its source—whether it is from grains, vegetables, fresh fruit, dried fruit, nuts, seeds, or beans. A new study of French adults shows conclusively how important it is for us to get our fiber from a variety of these sources. The study shows that when we eat fiber from grains we are likely to have a lower BMI, lower blood pressure, and less homocysteine, which is a risk factor for heart disease. Fiber from vegetables also leads to lower blood pressure and homocysteine, but not to a lower BMI. Fiber from fruit is also associated with lower blood pressure, but in addition, it has a positive connection with a lower waist-to-hip ratio. Dried fruit, nuts, and seeds contain fiber. Of primary importance to people with diabetes is its positive association with lower blood glucose levels. But fiber from this source also has many other benefits, including lower BMI, waist-to-hip ratio, and fasting apo B levels. The least well-known of these terms is apo B. It occurs in low density lipoprotein (LDL), known familiarly as the bad cholesterol.

Everybody tells us that we have to stop eating so much of this and that, specifically starches, sugars, fat, and even protein. But there's one exception. Almost all of us need more fiber of all types and sources. Consider it a free food.

Is STEVIA OR SPLENDA BETTER FOR YOU?

Is it better to sweeten your food with Splenda, the McNeil Nutritionals brand of sucralose, or use one of the many brands of stevia? I keep changing my mind on this question and going back and forth between them. I suspect that I'm not the only one puzzling over this issue. I've just switched back to stevia. It wasn't because of any new information or sudden insight. It was partly because I have begun to accept that people and organizations I respect prefer stevia.

The natural foods store Whole Foods Market, where I buy almost everything else that I eat, doesn't sell Splenda. Andrew Weil, MD, the leading exponent of integrative medicine, prefers stevia to any of the artificial sweeteners. "The only non-caloric sweetener I recommend is stevia, an herb in the chrysanthemum family native to Paraguay," he writes. "Stevia is safe for diabetics and is widely used as a sweetener around the world, especially in Japan and Brazil." Most stevia now comes from China.

Stevia is indeed natural. But natural isn't necessarily safe. Think of all the poisonous mushrooms, to say nothing of strychnine and curare. Eating poisonous mushrooms can cause liver failure and death. Strychnine, which comes from the seeds of a tree, kills from asphyxiation caused by paralysis of the pathways that control breathing or by exhaustion from convulsions. Curare, which comes from some plants grown in South America, kills by asphyxiation.

It's hard to determine the advantages and disadvantages of the natural stevia, which is essentially untested, against the artificial Splenda, which has been tested. But a tested and FDA-approved form of stevia may be coming. It's called rebiana. Coca-Cola and Cargill are working together to develop a refined formulation of stevia. Already, Coke has filed two dozen patent applications for it.

Splenda also doesn't compare with stevia in one respect that is important to people with diabetes. Splenda must have some glycemic value and some calories. That's because the manufacturers of Splenda (as well as the people who make aspartame) bulk up all retail forms of it with small amounts of maltodextrin, which is high glycemic. But no one has tested Splenda's glycemic value. Bulking up was what tricked me for a long time into thinking that Splenda must be a lot less expensive than stevia. But you use much less stevia to get the same amount of sweetness.

Stevia hasn't gone through the FDA's testing procedure, but stevia has been available as "a dietary supplement" ever since 1994. This strange law forbids the sale of stevia as a sweetener — the only thing that we use it for. That's why you won't find it in the same aisle as sugar and honey at Whole Foods, but rather in the areas where they sell vitamins, herbs, and such.

Because people in South American have used stevia for centuries and because many more in Japan, Korea, and China have used it for 20 years or so, many people argue that it must be safe. But it is not generally recognized as safe, or GRAS, the FDA's category for food ingredients like sugar that have been used so long that they predate premarket testing.

You can get stevia in three forms, and I've tried them all. The most natural and at the same time the least satisfactory is the powdered green leaf. It has a bitter aftertaste. You can buy stevia in liquid form, and some people might like to get it this way, but I don't. My preferred way, which I think is also the most common way, is a white extract of stevia.

I've tried all the major brands of stevia. Some of them do have a bitter aftertaste just like the raw leaf does. Right now, I prefer the Now Foods "Stevia Extract" and the NuNaturals "NuStevia," neither of which have a bitter aftertaste. Friends also recommend the KAL brand, but I haven't been able to find it.

PROFILE
GERI MATTILA QUIT SNACKING

Byetta is a tool that Geri Mattila uses to help her quit snacking. Slowly, it is helping her to lose weight and get her blood glucose numbers under control.

"People need to know that things happen, but maybe not as fast as we would like," she says "You have to put effort into it. It isn't a miracle weight loss cure. Slow but steady wins the race."

In her first 14 months on Byetta, Geri's weight is down from 226 pounds to 195 and she is still losing. Her A1C in that time is also down—from 8.6 to 7.3. So, too, are her morning numbers, down to the 120s and 130s, instead of the 160s and 170s; she says she feels that, finally, she has the **dawn phenomenon** under control.

Still, Splenda is clearly superior to stevia is one respect. You can cook with it. Stevia doesn't brown, crystallize, retain moisture, or make foods gooey. So don't expect me to throw out the Splenda that I have on hand now.

WHY YOU NEED ORGANIC FOOD

Not long ago, my friend Jeff Myers and I were discussing why it is important for people with diabetes to eat the highest-quality food. Jeff has type 1 diabetes and at the time was a diabetes life and wellness coach. He now works for the largest insulin pump company.

"Organic foods have a higher nutrient density," Jeff maintained. Until recently, we didn't have proof that organic produce was nutritionally superior. But several recent studies confirm Jeff's assertion. One study compared the same varieties of corn, strawberries, and blackberries grown on neighboring plots, but using organic or conventional methods. The researchers found that the organic fruits and vegetables had significantly higher levels of vitamin C and of several different polyphenols, which we now know have an important role in human health. Another study analyzed the government's nutrient data for 43 crops and how they changed between 1950 and 1999. The study found marked declines in six different nutrients and suggested that they were a trade-off for higher yields.

I'm sure that you will note that David's Diabetes Diet talks only about foods and includes only a single recipe. That's because the food choices are the basis of a diet. You can adapt any of your favorite recipes to reflect these sound eating principles.

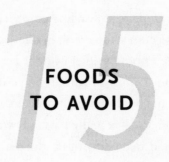

FOODS
TO AVOID

The easiest way to start eating less is to avoid empty calories and junk food. And doing this at home is a lot easier than when you eat at a fast-food place or even at most expensive restaurants.

YOU CAN COOK BETTER THAN THE CHEFS

So you can do a big favor to your health, to say nothing of your wealth, if you cut back on eating out. I would be surprised if the portions you or your spouse dishes up are anywhere near the size that those ever-so-helpful waiters will bring you in essentially all but the most avant-garde restaurants.

At home, you also have a lot more control over the ingredients of the foods you eat. Restaurants are beginning to let us know how many calories, grams of fat and sugar, and milligrams of sodium their dishes have—if we know where to look or whom to ask. My suspicious mind thinks that most of the time they don't want us to know because these levels are so high.

You Can Sweeten without Calories

The weight-loss benefits of avoiding empty calories from sugar and high-fructose corn syrup are straightforward. We can eliminate these calories from our diet without changing the taste of what we are eating simply by substituting a nonnutrient sweetener. While the major nonnutrient sweeteners—aspartame, sucralose, and saccharin—actually have a few calories, since the manufacturers add maltodextrin or glucose to bulk them up, this is usually in such a small amount that we can ignore them. Many people, however, use a noncaloric supplement called stevia as a sweetener. See the chapter on "Sugars" for more about controlling our sweet teeth.

Throw Out the Bad Fats

But some of what we call junk food may not be sweetened at all. The connection with weight loss isn't, then, quite as clear. But junk food high in saturated or trans fats is still junky and detrimental both to our health and to our weight loss. Avoiding junk food will reduce how much of these bad fats you eat. Saturated and trans fats are certainly bad fats. Not only do they play havoc with our cholesterol and triglyceride levels, they lead us into weight gain without any corresponding benefit that we can get from the good fats, those that are polyunsaturated, especially the omega-3s, and those that are monounsaturated.

All of the fats have far more calories than anything else, 9 per gram compared with 4 per gram for either protein or carbohydrates. Since fats are more energy dense than anything else that

PROFILE

BOB FARNWORTH IS NEVER HUNGRY

When Bob Farnsworth and I were initially in contact, he had lost 20 pounds in his first six weeks on Byetta. In the next year, he went on to lose another 16 pounds. He is down from a starting weight of 293 pounds to his current weight of 257. He has never had a weight gain except for a pound here or there, but rather a consistent loss.

His whole "relationship with food" changed. "I do not think about it," he says. "Never have I experienced going through a day without thinking of my next meal. Never have I eaten such controlled portions. The weight loss comes from a significant decrease in eating. Period. I am never hungry. I have had no nausea. In short, this drug is what I have been waiting for.

"I wonder, for those for whom the drug is not working, apart from a genetic answer, if the problem isn't desire. Many people for whom the drug is working were highly motivated prior to its use. They were serious about diet and exercise prior to beginning. Often, like me, they had fairly controlled blood glucose levels. But for those people with diabetes who are looking for a magic pill or shot to keep eating what they want, perhaps nothing works. I feel most sad for those experiencing great nausea. I have been lucky there, and it would be frustrating if I were a nausea victim who couldn't take Byetta. Even my morning numbers (always my worst in the past, from 130 to 150) have fallen for the first time to an average of 105. I love this drug. I believe it is the eating answer I have searched for. With some reports about long-term use potentially healing pancreatic function, it may be much more."

Bob had what he calls an interesting side effect of the Byetta. "Shortly after an injection one day I came down the stairs to the smell of my wife cooking one of my favorite foods—bacon. The smell of the grease with the recent injection made me queasy. I have been unable to eat bacon for over a year. And I once loved it. Weird stuff, this "better living through chemistry!"

we can eat, when we are trying to lose weight, it makes sense to avoid the bad ones as much as possible and go easy even on the good ones. See the chapter on "Bad Fats" for more on this heavy subject. Extra-virgin olive oil, avocados, nuts, and seeds are all great foods, but eating a lot of any of these good fats will still work against our weight-loss efforts.

You Can Kick the Salt Habit

Beyond avoiding bad sweeteners and bad fats, almost all of us need to cut way back on the salt in our food or the salt that we add at the table. The connection between salt and weight is not as direct as that of the other two prime nutritional demons. But too much salt leads to high blood pressure in some people, which is a real danger to our hearts.

Also, the more salt we eat, the more water we retain, so the heavier we become. While some people say this is "just water," the more salt we eat also makes us hungrier for ever more salty food. Ever eat just one salty potato chip or corn chip?

Just eliminating those foods sweetened with sugar or high-fructose corn syrup, those high in saturated fats or any added trans fats, and those high in salt can make your shopping expeditions go a lot faster. You have just ruled out perhaps 90 percent of all the stuff that your friendly neighborhood supermarket carries. You can now bypass acres of supermarket aisles.

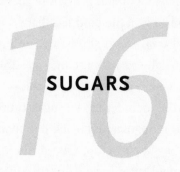

SUGARS

Avoid sugar? But the American Diabetes Association has been saying for years that people with diabetes can eat sugar! Certainly. A little sugar now and then won't spike your blood glucose. But if you want to lose weight, it will add calories that you simply don't need.

You Can Take Sugar Off the Table

Let's be a little technical here. When I talk about sugar, I mean sucrose. That's the real name for table sugar, which is highly processed sucrose, usually from sugar cane or sugar beets. I am not talking about other sugars, like the fructose and lactose occurring naturally in foods such as fruit and milk. Even vegetables and meat contain some sugar. They aren't a problem. It goes without saying, I hope, that we already minimize the sugars that are even higher-glycemic, maltose and glucose. Maltose, more commonly called malt sugar, works the quickest to spike our blood. Glucose, the primary sugar in corn syrup, is not far behind. And dextrose is the same as glucose.

Eliminating added sucrose is possible, although it takes a little knowledge and a lot of doing. Sucrose goes by a lot of names on the nutrition labels of the products that we buy in supermarkets and natural food stores. Probably no ingredient is more ubiquitous or goes by so many names as sugar. What we call sugar—whether white, granulated, or table—is only the tip of the crystal. Sucrose includes brown sugar, turbinado sugar, and most of the sugar in regular and blackstrap molasses and almost all of the sugar in maple syrup. One of the trickiest names is "organic dehydrated cane juice." I'm sure that it fools a lot of people into thinking they aren't getting sugar. Sucanat is another name for dried sugarcane juice. So-called raw sugar includes demerara, muscovado, and turbinado. More than 100 different sucrose substances exist. Adding sugar to food often does enhance its taste. But the cost is too high, not only in terms of rotting teeth but in boosting calories.

YOU CAN TAKE SUGAR TO A HIGHER LEVEL

One other sugar is probably even worse for us than sucrose, glucose, or maltose. I mean high-fructose corn syrup, not to be confused with plain fructose, which surely is a strange sugar. Fructose is the sweetest natural sugar, yet it has the lowest glycemic value of any sugar. Nutritionists often recommend that people with diabetes use fructose. Many of our favorite fruits and vegetables get their sweetness from fructose. We love honey, tree fruits, berries, and melons because of the fructose they have. Vegetables such as beets, sweet potatoes, parsnips, and onions are also loaded with fructose. And yet, many people

link our increased consumption of fructose to the national obesity epidemic. Generally, these people aren't talking about the
fructose in fruits and vegetables. Most of them are concerned
about the fructose in high-fructose corn syrup, which we are
consuming more and more of, particularly in soft drinks.

CAN YOU ENJOY FRUIT FRUCTOSE?

Some people also rail against fructose in any form—including that
in fruit. That's an extreme position. But even scientists and the
American Diabetes Association warn that fructose can increase

---

PROFILE
FRANCES ROUSE ALLOWS DAILY SWEETS

"I watch every bite of food that goes in my mouth," Frances
Rouse says. "Eating frequent small meals helps a great deal."

In her first three months on Byetta she has lost 18 pounds, with
60 more pounds to go. She considers that slow progress. "I've always had a tough time losing weight, so I'm not surprised it is
slow in coming off. In contrast, I've lost lots of inches."

She says that her "blood glucose is in the normal range." Her
early morning fasting level has not been over 110.

Frances's meal plan allows for daily sweets such as ice cream or
a cookie. She uses a food log and blood glucose records to tell her
which foods spike her levels. For her, an apple causes such a spike.
Her weight loss is steady and continues in spite of her "dietary
lapses," which she knows all of us have.

"My goal is to keep all of my pieces and parts attached to me
and in working order. I'm very pleased with the results. Thank you,
Byetta!"

cholesterol levels. "Fructose may adversely affect plasma lipids," the ADA says. "Therefore, the use of added fructose as a sweetening agent is not recommended; however, there is no reason to recommend that people with diabetes avoid naturally occurring fructose in fruits, vegetables, and other foods."

John P. Bantle, MD, has published the most knowledgeable and professional review of the pros and cons of using fructose. He is a professor of medicine in the division of endocrinology and diabetes at the University of Minnesota. It was largely his earlier research that prompted the ADA to recommend against our using added fructose. For some reason that we don't fully understand, fructose is particularly bad for the cholesterol levels of men.

That's clear. But what about the fructose in fruits and vegetables? Should we worry? Dr. Bantle says no. "Fructose that occurs naturally in fruits and vegetables is a modest component of energy intake and should not be of concern," he writes in his new article. The conclusion reads, "Adding large amounts of fructose to the diet may be undesirable. Nevertheless, concern about fructose should not extend to the naturally occurring fructose in fruits and vegetables. These are healthy foods which provide only a modest amount of fructose in most diets."

Dr. Bantle's conclusion is a logical one. Richard Carlson had the same idea in his best-seller *Don't Sweat the Small Stuff*. And as far back as the Romans, clear thinkers have argued that we should not bother with trifles. The concept is even embodied in American law. Many years ago I was a foreign service officer working for the U.S. Agency for International Development, America's foreign aid program. I still remember how our staff lawyers used a legal concept that they called "de minimis." It comes from a Latin phrase that means that the law is not interested in trivial matters. For the rest of my life I have dismissed trivialities as de minimis. Likewise, I hereby dismiss any concern about the fructose in fruits and vegetables as de minimis.

17

BAD
FATS

Some people think that all fats are bad for you. But the experts know that some fats are good for you and some are worse than others. Fats go by many different names. But we need to avoid just two of them as much as we can—saturated and trans fats.

Skip the Saturated Stuff

Saturated fat is the biggest culprit in raising total and LDL cholesterol levels. While it seems counterintuitive, it is the saturated fat, and not the cholesterol that we eat, such as that in eggs, that causes us to have high total and LDL cholesterol levels. "Dietary cholesterol has relatively little effect on blood cholesterol," is the conclusion of a review article in *The Journal of Nutrition, Health and Aging.*

Eating a lot of saturated fat leads to hardening of the arteries, cardiovascular disease, and heart disease: "There appears to be a consistent positive association of cholesterol, saturated fat, and possibly trans-fatty acid intake and atherosclerotic disease [hardening of the arteries]," according to a review article in *Cardiology Clinics* journal.

"Saturated fat reduction is a primary goal for decreasing the risk of cardiovascular disease," according to a recent review in *Nutrition Reviews*.

"Epidemiological studies have confirmed a strong association between fat intake, especially saturated and trans fatty acids, plasma cholesterol levels and rate of coronary heart disease (CHD) mortality," according to yet another medical researcher.

People with diabetes already have one of the risk factors for heart disease. If we are overweight, that makes two. We don't need to collect any more risk factors.

Fat occurs naturally in most of the foods we eat. This fat varies in its proportion of saturated and unsaturated fat. Foods that contain a high proportion of saturated fat include meat, butter and other dairy products, especially cream, ice cream, and cheese; coconut, cottonseed and palm kernel oil; meat; and many prepared foods. Dr. Robert Atkins, the pied piper of low carb, would rather have you drink cream than milk, because cream has almost no carbohydrates. But cream has more saturated fat than anything else. Only some cheeses come close. Ever hear about "pork, the other white meat"? That's what pork producers call it. It might be lean by some standards, but pork products—especially bacon and pork ribs—are some of the foods highest in saturated fat after cream and cheese. Even beef ribs don't have as much saturated fat as bacon and pork spareribs.

"Lower saturated fat to under 7 percent of calories (about 17 grams)," the *Harvard Health Letter* recommends in its April 2007 issue. But following that advice would be awfully difficult if you eat meat and dairy products. Just one pork spare rib has 20 grams of saturated fat. Just 3 ounces of cheddar cheese or one-third of a cup of cream has 18 grams of saturated fat. If we all became vegetarians, we wouldn't have any problem with saturated fat that we eat. I'm not advocating that we go that far, and I haven't gone that far myself. But I have eliminated beef, pork, butter, cheese, milk, and cream from my diet. The only dairy product that I continue to enjoy is yogurt, and then only when I can get it plain and nonfat.

Bison, sometimes but incorrectly known as buffalo, is much lower in saturated fat than beef. I find it to be even more tasty, as long as I don't overcook it. Chicken and fish also provide lots of protein and little saturated fat. I now completely avoid both butter and margarine. Instead, I use Spectrum Spread, which has no trans fat and only one-half gram of saturated fat per tablespoon. While few supermarkets and natural food stores carry it, they generally have other spreads that have no trans fat and only a gram of saturated fat per tablespoon. The hardest thing for me to find was anything that can substitute for cheese. But some almond or rice cheese, available in natural food stores, is both tasty and healthful.

DON'T TAKE THE TERRIBLE TRANS

Most nutritionists think that trans fat is even worse for us than saturated fat. Careful studies show that trans fat raises the bad LDL cholesterol and substantially lowers the good HDL cholesterol. It has other effects that lead to clogged arteries that in turn result in more heart disease.

Only in 2006 was the FDA able to require that manufacturers add trans fat contents to the nutrition facts label. Back in 1999 the FDA proposed including the amount of trans fat on the nutrition label. But then the agency waited for the Institute of Medicine of the National Academy of Sciences to complete its study so that it could set a daily value and upper limit for trans fat. The institute released its report in 2002. It recommended that we keep our trans fatty acid consumption as low as possible, because "there is a positive linear trend between trans fatty acid intake and total and LDL cholesterol concentration." Consumption of trans fatty acid, therefore, increases the risk of heart disease, the institute's report says.

This suggests that the upper limit of trans fat should be zero, the report continued. About 95 percent of trans fat in our diet comes from partially hydrogenated vegetable oil, which we can eliminate from our diet. But meat and dairy products have some natural trans fat, and eliminating them from our diet would require "extraordinary changes" that could lead to our getting too little protein and certain micronutrients. Consequently, the institute did not propose an upper limit. And since it did not give an upper level or reference daily intake, the FDA couldn't set a daily value for trans fat.

Because trans fat, like saturated fat, is linked to heart disease, the new label is especially relevant to people with diabetes. According to the Centers for Disease Control and Prevention, "Heart disease is the leading cause of diabetes-related deaths. Adults with diabetes have heart disease death rates about 2 to 4 times higher than adults without diabetes." Trans fat consumption is also associated with the risk of getting type 2 diabetes in the first place. The *American Journal of Clinical Nutrition* in 2001 reported a study that took a new look at the amount and types of fat that 84,204 women ate over a 14-year period and how many of them got type 2 diabetes. The study found no association between total fat, saturated fat, or monounsaturated fat and the risk of type 2 diabetes. Polyunsaturated fat reduced the risk. Only trans fat increased the risk of type 2 diabetes among the women studied.

PROFILE
TRACEY SMITH CAN'T EAT HIGH-FAT FOODS

Tracey Smith lost around 40 pounds on metformin after her doctor diagnosed her with diabetes in May 2006. But her blood glucose levels were still more than 250 each morning. "I was eating almost nothing and getting very frustrated with my levels," she says. When her doctor suggested Byetta, her morning blood glucose levels dropped almost 100 points. She says that on Byetta she has lost 20 more pounds and that she also experiences "the very full, no cravings effect, with very little nausea." Tracey is a teacher who expects to lose even more weight during summer vacation, when she increases her activity level.

"I think that the Byetta has helped to curb my appetite tremendously," she says. "I certainly can't eat as much as I did before, and certain foods make me feel horrible. Luckily, those are the 'bad for me' kinds of foods—those that are high in fat."

"I feel better than I have in months and am excited to see what the future holds," she concludes. "I still have quite a bit of weight to lose and hope that the meds continue working their little miracles, as well as keeping my sugar under control. It is very possible that having diabetes has, ironically, saved my life."

About 40 percent of supermarket foods contain trans fat. The FDA said a few years ago that it's in 95 percent of cookies, 80 percent of frozen breakfast foods, 75 percent of salty snacks and chips, 70 percent of cake mixes, and almost half of all cereals. The products that it lists with the most trans fat include vegetable shortening, doughnuts, stick margarine, french fries, and microwaved popcorn.

The terms "trans fat" and "partially hydrogenated" mean the same thing, right? If that's true—and it is—how come some nutrition facts labels say that a product has no trans fat, while the ingredients list on the same product say that it has some "partially hydrogenated" oil? It took me a while to figure this one out. It's because of a little loophole. The FDA allows companies to claim that a product has no trans fat if the serving size has less than half a gram of it. And those half grams can add up. Personally, I refuse to eat anything that has the words "partially hydrogenated" in the ingredients list, even if the nutrition label claims that it has no trans fats.

By eliminating all added trans fats from your diet and severely restricting saturated fat, you can reduce your cholesterol levels dramatically. Do you want to have cholesterol levels within the normal range? Silly question. I could have just asked whether you want to have a heart attack.

18

TIPS FOR
WEIGHT LOSS

All my life I've been a fast eater. I tell myself that's because I don't like my food to cool down too much. I might not walk too fast, but I can usually beat everyone to the finish line of the meal.

WE CAN EAT SLOWER

It's important to slow down at the table. The trouble with eating fast is that when we don't slow down over our food, we can be full before we know it. When we eat fast, we can eat more than we need to satisfy our hunger. Everyone knows that bit of conventional wisdom. But we didn't have any proof of it until October 2006, when researchers at the University of Rhode Island reported on "Eating Rate and Satiation." They compared how much people ate when they gobbled down their food and when they savored their meal. The people who ate more slowly not only took in fewer calories but also had a greater feeling of satiety both when they had just finished and also an hour later.

They even said that they enjoyed the meal more than when they were in the quick-eating group.

WE CAN BE MORE MINDFUL OF WHAT WE EAT

Some of my best weight-loss tips come from Brian Wansink, the director of Cornell University's Food and Brand Lab and the author of a 2006 book, *Mindless Eating*. Professor Wansink has spent 20 years studying the hidden cues that determine how we eat. He taught me that the best way for me to eat slower is to think about my meal as I eat it. In practice, what this means is not to think about something else that we are watching on TV, listening to on the radio, or reading in the newspaper. Brian calls that all-too-common way of consuming our meals "mindless eating."

In his book, Brian reports many experiments that his university laboratory conducted showing how we can eat less. Some of my other favorite tips are:

1. People who eat only at the kitchen or dining room table eat less. And this doesn't mean eating at the kitchen sink, as I used to do when I ate juicy fruit. Eating at the sink or from a container is, of course, more efficient than putting it on a dish or in a bowl, which you will have to wash later. That efficiency is, however, just another good reason to avoid it, as I write in the chapter "Inefficiency Is NEAT."
2. When we eat directly from a package we eat more. Until I read this, I made an exception for eating some of the plain nonfat yogurt that I love. No more.

3. The best part of a dessert is the first three bites. This
   means that I now buy smaller pieces of fruit than I used to
   buy.

THE SIZE OF YOUR SERVINGS MATTERS, TOO

Then, Brian shows us that size matters in more ways than one.
Two of these ways are that when we use smaller bowls and
smaller spoons we eat less. I eat a lot of stews and soups, but
now I use smaller bowls than I did before and I use teaspoons
rather than tablespoons or soup spoons. When I decide ahead
of time how big my portion will be, I am most successful at lim-
iting how much I eat for dinner. That decision needs an action
boost. I cook a lot of stews and chili bean dishes, always making
enough in a big pot for several days. Typically, the first time I
have one of these delicious meals I eat a couple of bowlfuls. Because it's there. But on succeeding days, I take out just one serving, reheat it in the microwave, and immediately put the big pot
back in the refrigerator. That action leads me to stop with the
first bowl, no matter how good it tastes. An even more powerful
action is to freeze leftovers in meal-size portions and take one
portion out of the freezer well before dinner. That way, you
really have a long wait to get seconds!

At a minimum, I wait at least 10 minutes after finishing my
serving before taking a second helping. Often, I even go as far
as to set the kitchen timer to give me an external cue to wait
long enough. By then, I almost always feel full and don't want
any more.

You Can Keep Track

Just increasing the awareness of what you eat can help you to eat less. Another man who is consulting on a Joslin Diabetes Center project with me says that he lost more than 100 pounds in a couple of years by taking a digital photograph of everything he ate. He says that he doesn't even look at the photographs after taking them, but the act of recording what he eats helps him to stay in control. Others are able to achieve the same results by keeping a food log. I kept a log recording all the calories and available carbohydrates—sugars and starches, but not fiber—that I ate for a couple of months. It takes a little effort, but it was worth it to get a hang of whether I was eating too much or not enough. "It's annoying and it's tedious" to count calories and keep a diary recording what you eat and when you eat it, a dieter named Ron Krauss told Gina Kolata, author of *Rethinking Thin*. But that's precisely the point. "It is a disincentive to eat when you have to look everything up and find its calories and weigh it and write it down. Sometimes I'd just as soon not eat," he said.

When you keep a food log, you need a source of reliable calorie and carbohydrate data. If you have an Internet connection, a quick and reliable source is the U.S. Department of Agriculture's Web site for the National Nutrient Database, www.nal.usda.gov/fnic/foodcomp/search/. Otherwise, you can use Corinne T. Netzer's *Complete Book of Food Counts*, which is now in its 7th edition. A handy alternative is a pocket-size electronic calorie counter called the Track3 made by Coheso, a company in Pleasanton, California. It lets us look up nutritional information for more than 35,000 foods, including 250 restaurants and 500 food brands. It can calculate nutrition content, including calories, carbohydrates, fiber, protein, fat, and sodium for individual foods and for recipes. It also lets us add 1,000 new food items and meals and personal exercise information as well as letting us create a handy list of favorite foods. The Track3 also lets us keep track of not only the calories we consume, but also how many we burn when we exercise. We can also use it to log our blood glucose readings and the insulins or oral medications that we take.

YOU CAN AVOID TEMPTATION

One of the hardest dietary lessons for me to learn is something that I don't remember ever seeing in writing. Maybe it can help others. I don't buy anything that I just can't stop eating or drinking, even when I am on Byetta. What's irresistible to me may not be for you. But I just can't have chocolates, ice cream, kefir, cheese, nut butters, chips, or bread around me without eating it all. If I ever eat any of these delicious temptations, it will not be where I live! So I limit myself to eating just a bit of what other people offer me in their homes or as free samples in food stores. I can control myself there, because I would be ashamed to eat their entire stash.

Avoid especially the all-you-can-eat restaurants. My nemesis is the buffet at Indian restaurants, because I love Indian food so much. Nowadays, I avoid the all-you-can-eat buffet restaurants, remembering that quality is better for me than quantity.

In a similar vein, Tara Parker-Pope, the weekly health columnist and reporter for *The Wall Street Journal*, suggests that we downsize our favorite foods. "We all have favorite foods we eat almost every day," she writes. "Instead of giving them up, look for ways to trim calories." The best way to stay in control of what you eat is to prepare it yourself. Parker-Pope points out that restaurant and take-out foods have far more saturated fat, calories, and sodium than foods that you cook in your own kitchen. "One way to cut calories is simply to commit to home cooking more often," she writes. "Studies show a direct relationship between cooking at home and body mass index. In the past 30 years, every half hour less we spent preparing food at home, body mass index increased by 0.5."

In restaurants, fast or slow, these days they almost universally serve you huge portions. So when you go out to eat with your spouse or a good friend, it's a good idea to order one entrée and two plates so that you can share the meal. You can also ask your waiter to put a part of it in a doggy bag. Some people even suggest that you ask your waiter ahead of time to do that, so that you don't even face the temptation of that huge portion.

Likewise, consider not snacking on some days. I know that whenever I start eating, I want to keep going. So at least for me sometimes the best way to avoid overeating is not to start, except at regular meals. Even with Byetta, it's easiest to stay away from the temptation. The only such exceptions that I make are when I absolutely need a sweet. Then I eat a piece of fruit or suck on a Ricola sugar-free throat drop. A medium apple has about 70 calories. But two of these throat drops have only 17 calories.

YOU CAN LOSE WEIGHT BY EATING

The really good news is that eating breakfast can actually help you lose weight. A new study shows that breakfast skippers were heavier than those who ate breakfast. Before breakfast is the best time to weigh yourself. I make sure to weigh and record the results the first thing each morning. I prefer scales that have a digital readout to those that are **analog**, because I can't interpret—and perhaps fudge—the digital result.

WHEN DO YOU WANT TO WEIGH?

But be forewarned that your weight will go up and down for unfathomable reasons, cautions my friend John Dodson. Don't let it discourage you when you have done everything right the day before and your weight still goes up. Because weight loss on a daily basis is unpredictable, many experts recommend weighing yourself only once a week or so. That makes a lot of sense, and I used to do that. But I think that weighing myself every day makes even more sense, because is the only way to get the immediate knowledge that I need to control what and how much I eat.

YOUR AFTER-DINNER DANGERS

The worst time to eat is after dinner. What we eat then doesn't have a chance to get digested while we are still at least relatively active. I *always* ate after dinner before going to bed—and sometimes even afterward. When I started taking Byetta, this habit continued for a while but eventually dropped away.

Your Waste, Not Your Waist

Make it a point sometimes to leave something on your plate — even if you waste it. You don't have to eat everything that's there, even if your mother kept telling you about all the starving children in China and India. If you can leave something to be eaten another day or not at all, you are in control.

PROFILE
Lance Brofman Doesn't Finish His Meals

Before Lance started taking Byetta, if he didn't eat everything on his plate when he went to a restaurant, he "would feel depressed (or maybe deprived is a better word) about not eating that last bit." Now he feels good about not eating everything, possibly because overeating on Byetta tends to bring on gastronomic distress.

When he started taking Byetta, he weighed 272 pounds, and his A1C was 6.5. Ten months later, he weighed 203, and his A1C is down to 5.7.

Lance had previously lost some weight on the South Beach Diet. But he gained it all back. He had also previously been taking Avandia and one of the sulfonylureas but stopped taking both diabetes medications the day after he started Byetta.

He never experienced nausea on Byetta. But, he says, what he perceives as satiety, others may think of as nausea.

It seems that everything we do relates somehow to our weight. Even sleeping. If we don't get enough sleep, many of us try to give our energy a boost by snacking. While that will temporarily help us to repay our sleep debt, it will make us gain weight.

The National Weight Control Registry tracks more than 5,000 people who have succeeded in keeping their weight off for a long time. The *Mayo Clinic Health Letter* studied these biggest losers in its January 2007 issue. As the article shows, different strategies work for different people, and nothing works all of the time. But the most common motivation of the losers who succeeded was concern over their health or coming to the realization that their weight was at an all-time high. Those were my motivations in spades. What are yours?

INEFFICIENCY IS NEAT
Why You Need to Waste Effort

Even those people who can't stand the thought of working out every day have one way of using their energy. It is literally what they do every day whether or not they want to or even think about it. It's just that many of us are so efficient that we don't do enough. If you are as efficient as I am, you might be in trouble. I know I was.

HOW YOU CAN SAVE TIME, LOSE BODY

Why would anyone want to be anything except as efficient as possible? With all the things that we have to do every day, we couldn't get them all done unless we managed them with time-saving strategies. Unfortunately, we can be too efficient for our own good. We can take care of everything out there in the world except our own bodies. It's not surprising that people who are especially efficient physically are often overweight and have diabetes as well. We may forget that the routines of daily life are a way that we use energy, just like walking, swimming, and lifting weights. It's only when we use more energy than we take in that we lose weight.

You might think, as I once did, that apparently dumb things like fidgeting, tapping your foot, and forgetting to do your chores in as few steps as possible are a simple waste of effort. But Dr. James Levine, a Mayo Clinic endocrinologist and nutritionist, calls this *non*exercise *a*ctivity *t*hermogenesis, or NEAT. Dr. Levine and his associates described their findings in a 2005 issue of *Science*. But for us, his talk with Denise Grady of The *New York Times* was much more interesting than the technical report. "People with obesity are tremendously efficient," Dr. Levine told her. "Any opportunity not to waste energy, they take. If you think about it that way, it all makes sense. As soon as they have an opportunity to sit down and not waste those calories, they do."

How You Can Become Inefficient

That was me in spades. Before reading this, I prided myself on not wasting effort. I have now become physically inefficient, but it wasn't easy. Nevertheless, ever since reading Dr. Levine's research, I have become less efficient. And every time I do something inefficiently instead of mentally beating myself over the head for it, as I did before, I am now just pleased that I can take a few more steps than I otherwise would. Not only do I get a bit more exercise this way, but, even more profound, this tip from Dr. Levine had as positive an effect on my mental health as any I have ever read.

The doctor practices what he preaches. The study's findings inspired him to redesign his office. He mounted his computer over a treadmill, and while he works, he is walking at the rate of 0.7 miles per hour. "I converted a completely sedentary job to a mobile one," he said. He says that he actually enjoys working at his computer now. There's no way that I could put my desktop computer on my treadmill. Even my new laptop doesn't fit securely enough. Instead, I borrow books on CDs from my local library, copy them to my iPod, and listen to them whenever I get on the treadmill. Lately, I have listened to more books than I've read. It's okay to be efficient while exercising, isn't it?

20

AEROBIC EXERCISE

Three things help you control type 2 diabetes. The easiest is taking the medication your doctor prescribes. The hardest is your diet, because of the never-ending decisions about what, how much, and when to eat. Exercise comes between these extremes, and the easiest way to start exercising is simply to walk more. Walking is the prime example of aerobic exercise. This is one example of one type of exercise that we need to do regularly to be healthy. The next chapter looks at the other type, resistance training.

YOUR EXERCISE PRESCRIPTION

More and more doctors recognize that exercise is good medicine. Someone wrote recently that prescribing exercise along with medication is the coming thing. It isn't—it's already here. Dr. Richard K. Bernstein, an endocrinologist in Mamaroneck, New York, wrote *Dr. Bernstein's Diabetes Solution* and is known as the leading low-carb advocate for people with diabetes. He told me that he already prescribes specific exercise to most of his patients. Another endocrinologist who regularly prescribes exercise is Dr. Alan Rubin, author of *Diabetes for Dummies*.

A recent meta-analysis studied the 14 randomized controlled trials comparing people with type 2 diabetes who got exercise with those who didn't. The conclusion: Exercise improves blood glucose control and decreases body fat content for people with type 2 diabetes.

Exercise makes you feel and look better. It reduces your stress. It takes glucose out of your blood to use for energy. It helps prevent heart disease, depression, and even some forms of cancer. If you do enough, it will help you to lose weight.

Being physically inactive is one risk factor for heart disease; diabetes is another. Once you have diabetes you have to live with it, but you can reverse inactivity.

A common recommendation is for your doctor to examine you before you start an exercise program. Certainly, a doctor should check out people with diabetic eye disease and blood vessel problems. But since it could be an excuse to postpone exercise, I wondered if everyone needs a checkup. "I do think that the eye and vascular condition would warrant a special bit of advice," Dr. Joe Prendergast told me. "But the rest would not." Dr. Rubin also tends to agree. "We all do some walking already," he told me. "If all you are doing is walking, I don't think an exam is necessary. The important thing is to start at a low level and build up. But if you want to go from a sedentary lifestyle to vigorous exercise like mountain biking, jogging, or long distance running, it's a good idea to get a physician's okay."

WHEN YOU SHOULDN'T EXERCISE

People with type 1 diabetes, according to the American Diabetes Association's current position statement on exercise, should avoid exercise if their levels are more than 250 mg/dl (13.8 **mmol/L**) and they have ketosis—high levels of acidic substances called ketones—in their blood. They also shouldn't exercise if their level is over 300, even if they don't have ketosis. Even for people with type 2 diabetes, these are good cutoff levels to keep in mind.

Before strenuous exercise, it's also a good idea to measure your blood glucose and check your feet for cuts or blisters. During exercise, stop immediately and take three glucose tabs if you feel an insulin reaction coming on. After exercising, check your blood glucose level and feet again. Take a big drink of water before exercising. A water bottle on your treadmill or in your fanny pack or day pack also makes sense.

When you start exercising, you need a good pair of shoes. For walking, don't wear running, tennis, or basketball shoes, because they don't give you enough stability. Walking or cross-training shoes give you more lateral support than other sport shoes. Try on different shoes at a well-stocked store. Flex your feet, wiggle your toes, and walk around until you find a pair that feels comfortable. Never count on breaking in uncomfortable shoes.

On the trails, I am continually dismayed when I see other hikers who aren't using a walking staff or a pair of poles. I am so used to using them—particularly when going up or down a steep hill—that I can't imagine hiking without one. Yet, few hikers have caught on to the wisdom of this little appendage. People who are overweight or out of shape can benefit the most from them. And anyone who has used them to avoid a serious fall—as I have many times—know that they are worth every dollar they cost. Walking staffs and particularly a pair of poles improve our balance on uneven ground, reduce the stress on our joints and spine, and help us to walk more upright. They can be useful to ward off dogs (as I have more than once) or bears or mountain lions (I haven't yet had that opportunity). They also let us use our upper-body muscles and take the weight off our legs. When we use a walking stick or poles, we can take up to 20 percent of our weight from our lower body as we walk. Particularly if you have bad hips or an arthritic knee, this can make all the difference between walking and staying on the couch.

For about 20 years, my walking staff was a bamboo pole that had come with a rug wrapped around it. With a crutch tip on the end to avoid slipping and clattering, it was light in weight and completely satisfactory until the bamboo began to crack. Then, I switched to an even lighter aluminum walking staff. Recently, however I have doubled my assist. I got a pair of poles from a German company called Leki. But three U.S. firms— Black Diamond Equipment, Fittrek, and Exerstrider—as well as Finland's Excel and Norway's Swix Sport, which pioneered the activity in Europe, also offer a large selection of poles. Sometimes called trekking poles, sometimes Nordic walkers, and sometimes fitness walking poles, they are similar. By whatever name, they all make walking and hiking easier and safer.

PROFILE

CAROLE GONZALEZ THREATENED TO FIRE HER DOCTOR

"My health at age 65 was bad and I was clearly on the downhill slippery slope," Carole Gonzalez says. "I had to rock to get out of chairs and take a great deal of care not to sit where I could not get up on my own or have help. When I stood up, it took a while to unfold. I was also exhausted all the time and could only walk slowly. But my arms and face were pruning up nicely."

When she asked her doctor to prescribe Byetta, he refused. "So I threatened to fire him," Carole relates. "So, a year ago he prescribed it. He has seen too many yo-yo dieters to get all excited about weight loss since then, but in his own restrained way he has been excited to see mine. Plus, my most recent A1C two weeks ago was 6.5, and that did perk him up." Before she started to take Byetta, her A1C level had reached 9.8.

Carole weighed 236 on her bathroom scale when she started taking Byetta. A year later, she is down to 185 on the same scale. But she has been stuck there for several months. "So, I am going to have to get my food intake under better control," she says. "There is a big difference between knowing what not to eat and steadfastly refusing to give in to temptation."

Six months after starting Byetta, Carole began taking long walks. At first, it was just to the corner and back. Then, around the block. Now, she walks 3 $\frac{1}{2}$ miles every day before work and 5 miles on weekends. "Last week it was 27 miles, and two hours dancing." Now, she is ready to walk on uneven ground and for some form of resistance training. At 68, she knows that she has to be careful not to break or tear anything. So now she's going to try walking on the grass in the parks while carrying 3-pound weights to get used to the uneven surfaces. "We are talking baby steps here," she says. "I'll be the weird lady waving jaw breakers at dawn. Every neighborhood needs one. Little change by little change, and I have become 'Ms. Fleet of Foot.'"

YOUR EXERCISE CHOICES

Walking or hiking is the exercise of choice for most people. But neuropathy or other problems can make walking difficult for some. They usually find that doing water aerobics or swimming laps is a great alternative.

But what if it's too hot or cold or wet outside or takes too long to get to a place you like? Stay home and use a treadmill, a stationary bike, or a stair stepper. A few years ago, the example of some other people with diabetes inspired me to buy a treadmill. I use it exclusively until it gets warm enough here for me to go back to my favorite trails.

EXERCISE CAN BE EASY AND ENJOYABLE

You know the old saying, "No pain, no gain." You can forget it. Your exercise program doesn't have to be hard. A major study determined that you cut your risk of heart disease even if you do only light to moderate walking. The amount of time is more important than your pace. It's the deed, not the speed. And you don't have to do it all in one fell swoop.

Some people are out of shape because they think exercise is boring. Forget that, too. The key is choosing something you enjoy. I think it's easiest to be excited about what I'm doing when I'm walking a trail. There's always something new, even if I have been down that path hundreds of times. Walking with a partner also keeps it interesting.

But even when you work out at home or in a fitness center, you can make time pass more quickly by reading a magazine, listening to music or a book on CD, or watching television. Alternatively, you can just use that time to clear your mind. Your exercise can simply be something you do for yourself on a busy day devoted to the needs of other people. But, paradoxically, by getting yourself in a better mood, it can help others, too.

Gadgets can make our daily workouts more interesting, too. Some people use pedometers to measure how far they walk. Others use heart rate monitors to make sure that their workouts aren't too easy or too hard.

CAN YOU GET TOO MUCH EXERCISE?

The controversy is how much exercise: 30, 60, or 90 minutes a day. In 1996, the Surgeon General set a low bar, recommending that we get enough exercise to use at least 1,000 calories a week. This works out to be about 30 minutes of moderate physical activity on three or four days of the week. However, the government's current recommendation is that we get up to 90 minutes of exercise most days of the week. That's a lot more. I wondered whether the new recommendation asks so much that many of us will just throw up our hands and sit on our behinds. Dr. Prendergast told me that he thinks we will. He quoted Voltaire, who long ago said the French equivalent of "the best is the enemy of the good."

But Dr. Rubin doesn't feel that the new government standards are out of line. "There was a time when we thought it was unrealistic to ask people to stop smoking. Personally, I do at least 90 minutes of exercise daily and feel great as a result," he told me. "The patients in my practice who do best with their diabetes are the ones who do the most exercise. Some of them told me it was impossible for them to lose weight. The only way I have been successful with them is when they have done several hours of exercise every day." He points out a 2004 study that shows that overweight people lose more weight the more they exercise — even without dieting.

I have noticed that after a two- or three-hour walk, I am actually less hungry than I normally am, and I eat less. That may be part of its weight-loss charm. I know the conventional wisdom is that exercise is supposed to make you hungry, but it sure doesn't work that way for me.

We need a new mind-set. Our ancestors didn't call it exercise, but they walked for hours as they hunted for food. We no longer have to move around on our feet, so we invented something called exercise. When it becomes second nature to move around like our ancestors did, we begin to control our diabetes.

21
RESISTANCE IS
USEFUL

The Borg in the *Star Trek* fictional universe may have told you that "resistance is futile." That's not true. In fact, resistance can be good for your weight and overall health and can go a long way toward helping you to control your diabetes. Specifically, what I mean is **resistance training**. It goes by lots of other names, too, including strength training, weight training, and anaerobic exercise. The latter means "without oxygen." Whatever you call it, this type of exercise will increase your strength, muscular endurance, and muscle size. This is something that aerobic exercises like walking and working out on a treadmill won't do.

You Can Start at Home

Some people think that you've got to have special equipment, some knowledge of exercise techniques, and even personal instruction to do resistance training. Those are all good ideas as you get into it. But you certainly can get started without even going to a gym. "You can do it in your home," says Dr. Karl Knopf, a 54-year-old author and professor of adaptive physical education at Foothill College in Los Altos, California. He is also the founder and president of the Fitness Educators of Older Adults Association, a training and accreditation program. "Lift a rock or a can of beans," he told Kristi Essick, who interviewed him for *The Wall Street Journal*. It's all about repetitions. He says that to build strength it's best to start with six repetitions, and when you can do that many without much strain, build up to 15 repetitions.

You Need to Start Slow

Still, you have to be careful when you start resistance training. "High-resistance exercise using weights may be acceptable for young individuals with diabetes, but not for older individuals or those with long-standing diabetes," the American Diabetes Association cautions in its position statement on "Physical Activity/ Exercise and Diabetes." The statement continues, "Moderate weight training programs that utilize light weights and high repetitions can be used for maintaining or enhancing upper body strength in nearly all patients with diabetes. . . . Data on the effects of resistance exercise are not available for type 2 diabetes, although early results in normal individuals and patients with type 1 disease suggest a beneficial effect."

That was true in 2002, when they last revised the position statement. But a new comprehensive review of the literature and a new meta-analysis clearly show that resistance training is indeed good for people with type 2 diabetes. Is anybody surprised? Both articles appeared in recent issues of *Diabetes Care*, the American Diabetes Association's premier professional journal. First came the review by Neil Eves and Ronald Plotnikoff, "Resistance Training and Type 2 Diabetes," in August 2006.

EXERCISE MAKES YOU MORE SENSITIVE

Several studies that Eves and Plotnikoff reviewed showed that resistance training enhances our sensitivity to insulin. The largest published study in this area showed that even resistance training of low to moderate intensity if performed for a year or more improved not only blood glucose levels but also cholesterol, blood pressure, and especially weight. That study, by Stefano Balducci of La Sapienza University in Rome, Italy, and his colleagues, looked at what happened to a group of men and women who did aerobic plus resistance training for a full year. The study assigned to that training program 62 people with type 2 diabetes who averaged about 61 years of age and were previously sedentary. A control group of 58 people continued what they were doing (or not doing). Those in the control group had no significant changes. But those who did the aerobic and resistance training exercises showed significant decreases in their BMI, fat mass, and waist circumference. They also had significantly better cholesterol and triglyceride numbers and blood pressure levels.

The meta-analysis in *Diabetes Care* looked at the effect of three forms of exercise—resistance training, aerobic exercise, and a combination of the two. The report by Neil Snowling and Will Hopkins concluded on the basis of a review of 27 studies

PROFILE
Jana Tronier Uses Nausea

It's not willpower that helped Jana Tronier to lose a lot of weight. It's been nausea. "Willpower to me was not that important," she says, "The Byetta pretty much took care of it, since if I ate too much or the wrong thing I would throw up. I hate throwing up, and my body and brain have learned by trial and error to stop eating, even though it tastes good. Nothing is worse than throwing up!"

Until she learned this, when Jana first started on Byetta she was nauseated all of the time. But she still burps a lot more than before. The nice thing, she says, is that now she can actually eat food high in carbohydrates. For more than a year before going on Byetta she followed the Atkins induction diet, which allowed her only 20 grams of carbohydrate a day. Still, her blood glucose levels were in the 300 to 400 range. "Now they are perfectly normal."

Before she went on the Byetta, Jana had been working with a personal trainer for over a year, but with only marginal results. She still works with her trainer once a week, doing weight training and cardio for an hour.

Jana is 37, married with children. Diagnosed with diabetes in 2004, initially she went on insulin, but it led to a weight gain of 30 pounds in one month. Before she started on Byetta, she says that she was in denial, with A1C levels as high as 11.7, a dress size of 14, and a weight of about 200, but was "afraid to step on the scales." Six months later, her A1C in the low 6's, she wears a size 7 dress, and her weight is down to 145.

"With my weight loss I am way more active and confident," Jana says. "I actually leave my house to go grocery shopping, instead of just sitting home and making my husband do it. I also do more things now with my kids and family. My life is so much better!"

that all of these three forms of exercise help us. They "have small to moderate beneficial effects on glucose control in type 2 diabetic patients and small beneficial effects on some related risk factors for complications of diabetes."

Despite recommendations that we engage in resistance training, few of us with type 2 diabetes do so. In a sample of 1,193 people, only 12 percent did weight training or performed activities that would increase muscular strength.

HOW YOU CAN EXERCISE QUICKLY

When I first thought about adding resistance training to the hours I spend almost every day in aerobic exercise by walking or hiking or using the treadmill, it did seem daunting. The good news, of course, is that it helps us to control our diabetes. The perhaps less obvious good news is that it doesn't really take that much time.

Push-ups, sit-ups, and squats are examples of resistance training exercises that don't require any equipment. But if you are as obsessed by efficiency as I am, you can get some simple equipment that won't take *any* of your precious time to use.

I got a couple of dumbbells, which I think was a pretty smart thing to do. At first I bought two 5-pound weights that I kept next to my easy chair and lifted whenever I watched a movie on TV. I know that it's not much, but it was a start. Soon, it got to be too easy for me to make 15 repetitions. So I upgraded to 10-pound weights and then to 15-pound weights. And when that becomes too easy, I intend to get something even harder, which I think will be an even smarter thing to do.

The American College of Sports Medicine, for example, recommends that we perform resistance training two or more days a week. They suggest that we do about 8 to 10 exercises of our major muscle groups for around 10 to 15 repetitions. The American Diabetes Association has a similar recommendation. "People with type 2 diabetes should be encouraged to perform resistance exercise three times a week, targeting all major muscle groups, progressing to three sets of 8 to 10 repetitions at a weight that cannot be lifted more than 8 to 10 times."

If we start slow, we can easily build up to that level in practically no time. This is a way to resist that is certainly not futile.

22
METABOLISM AND EXERCISE

The surest way to be thin is to have a fast metabolism. Some people are born with it. Most of us are not. If you are among the majority, you can still speed up your metabolism and burn food faster. Exercise is the best tool that we have to do that. For most people, exercise is a dirty word. But losing weight is a dirty subject, so we need to consider exercise along with it. Only 58 percent of adult Americans who don't have diabetes get even 30 minutes of moderate or vigorous exercise three or more times a week. It's significantly less for people with diabetes, just 39 percent of adult Americans who have diabetes.

YOUR STARVATION SET POINT

When we take off a lot of weight, our body compensates for what it sees as the threat of starvation. So, here again the question of being too efficient comes up. In this case, when we take off a lot of weight, our bodies process the food that we eat too efficiently. Our metabolism slows down. Our body uses the calories we give it more slowly. Our body tends to reach its set point between weight and energy expenditure. Scientists call this homeostasis.

Three Rockefeller University physicians, Rudolph L. Leibel, Michael Rosenbaum, and Jules Hirsch, provided the most famous demonstration of the set point theory. Academically, however, they didn't call it our set point. Instead, they referred to it as a compensatory metabolic process that resists the maintenance of new, lower, weight. They monitored the metabolic rates of research subjects whom they put on tight diets and exercise programs. When the volunteers got more food, their metabolic rates went way up. But when they got much less food, their metabolic rates fell, preserving the status quo.

The set point of our weight is why few of us keep off the weight that we go to so much trouble to lose. When we try to reduce our weight below the point that our body is naturally set to have, our bodies begin to slow down. Also, as we lose weight, not only is our resting metabolic rate decreased, our nonresting energy expenditure is less because we are moving around less mass, which takes less effort. To keep our weight below our natural set point means that we have to do at least two things:

1. We have to keep watching what we eat and continually eat less as our weight and metabolism go down.
2. We have to exercise regularly to keep our metabolism up to speed. Because physical activity increases our energy expenditure and counteracts the reduction in our total energy expenditure, it is a key component of any weight-loss program.

Your Time/Intensity Trade

Studies of people who are successful at keeping weight off show that they need to devote an hour to 90 minutes a day to physical activity. But the activity doesn't have to be high intensity. Walking and taking the stairs rather than the elevator can make the difference. But you can save time if your activity is high intensity. It's a trade-off between quantity and quality. Even 30 minutes a day of more intense exercise may be just as good in speeding up our metabolism as 90 minutes of exercise where we don't push ourselves. David E. Tanner, DO, my doctor in Boulder, Colorado, is also a high-intensity athlete. He recommends that we work out at 70 to 80 percent of our maximum heart rate to keep our metabolism up so that we can keep off the weight we lose.

Dr. Tanner recommends that we start by using a heart rate monitor. The first step is to calculate your maximum heart rate. This is the fastest that your heart can beat for one minute. The easiest calculation is to subtract your age from 220. Then, multiply the result by 0.7 and then by 0.8 to find out what 70 percent and 80 percent of your maximum heart rate is.

To get your weight below your natural set point and keep it off, you may have to do a third thing, too. You probably will have to take a GLP-1 mimetic that reduces your hunger. Just dieting and exercising is probably not enough to dampen the forces in our society and your own bodies that otherwise would make you regain the weight you lost.

Conclusion

You will be able to lose weight if you have type 2 diabetes and take Byetta or one of the forthcoming drugs that mimic the action of GLP-1. Even taking metformin helps some people to lose weight. You don't even need to follow a single one of my suggestions about what to eat or how much to exercise. That's a fact proven by the participants in the clinical trials of Byetta. The people who ran the trials told the participants that they shouldn't make any changes in their lifestyle. Still, those who tested Byetta for us typically lost weight. On the average, it was 6 pounds in 30 weeks.

But if you want to lose a substantial amount, you can do a lot better than they did just by following some of the simple tips in this book. With Byetta or with one of the other drugs in the GLP-1 class that will soon be available, major weight loss is easier for us than for anybody else ever.

Our demon is our appetite. It's not that we enjoy life too much, but we focus our lives too closely on food. Byetta and the other forthcoming GLP-1 mimetics reduce our appetite for food so we have a greater appetite for the other good things of life. This gives us greater energy, especially if we get greater exercise, which in turn gives us even more energy.

Too Many Tips for You?

I do make an awful lot of suggestions about food and exercise in this book. This got me worried. I reminded myself of a book I read a couple of years ago that focused on an amino acid supplement called arginine that seems to have the potential to reverse the buildup of plaque in the arteries, which causes most heart disease.

I take 5 grams of the stuff every day myself, not because of the book, but because of what I have learned from Dr. Joe Prendergast. The book apparently didn't have too much to say about arginine, because the author of that book went on and on about all the other stuff we should be taking along with it. It was daunting and discouraging to me. If arginine is so great, I wondered, why do I have to take all these other supplements, too? This is different. All the other stuff besides Byetta or the alternatives that I'm sure we will soon have is just dressing on the cake, so to speak. Eat and exercise as much or as little as you are easily persuaded to do. It does get easier as we break old habits. For example, I used Byetta for months before I was able to refrain from eating after dinner, although I knew better. But I eventually broke the habit, and I don't even have that urge any more.

Can You Lose Weight Without Drugs?

Everybody says that it's better to lose weight without drugs. But look in the mirror and all around you. Everybody has tried that. It doesn't work. Individually and collectively, we are getting heavier. We don't all live in the best of all possible worlds. In the real world that we live in, it's too hard to lose weight without drugs because our lives are too easy.

We're Lucky to Have Diabetes

We are a "fast-food nation" in the unforgettable words of the book of that name by Eric Schlosser and the movie that he and Richard Linklater made from that book. We are a lucky nation because we have such an abundance of food and such a wealth of devices to do almost all of our physical work for us. But most of us are likewise unlucky, since we fail to compensate for all the food we eat and the exercise we don't get. Still, people with type 2 diabetes are especially lucky compared to other people who are overweight. I'm serious. That's because we have medication tested and approved for us that will help us lose weight and that our health insurance plans will usually cover most of its cost.

You May Need to Eat More

Some weeks, I seem to be losing weight a little faster than I would like. A lot of people say that you can lose weight too fast. So I put on the brakes and eat a little more for a day or two. That doesn't at all mean that I eat junk food. Just a little more of the healthy foods that I discussed here in previous chapters. Being able to eat at much as I like is such a switch for me that I haven't gotten over it yet!

You Can Help Your Medication

Some of these medications, like Byetta and the other forthcoming GLP-1 mimetics, can help you lose a lot of weight. But they aren't miracle cures. You have to help them along. How? Simply by eating right and exercising enough. That's why this book includes several chapters on diet and exercise. These are the two other keystones of diabetes control.

I know that you can lose a lot of weight on Byetta. If you want to. That's the key. I do know that the weight that I lost is much more than what people usually lose on Byetta. Was I just lucky? I don't think so. It was more than luck. It was a knowledge of what to do and a plan to do it.

Byetta alone won't make you lose a lot of weight. And it's not even the old question of willpower, because it certainly doesn't take the same willpower that so many people say is what we lack when we are overweight or obese. Still, Byetta can help us lose a *lot* of weight only if we exert appropriate effort. We just need to know that we have to lose a lot of weight and act on that knowledge. That's what worked for me and what can work for you.

Please Write

That's what I hope to impart with this book. I would certainly be delighted to hear from you. Please e-mail me at: mendosa@ mendosa.com

I would love to include your stories in the next edition of this book.

How Will You Celebrate Success?

Before I started taking Byetta and got my weight under control, there were a lot of things that I couldn't do. Some of them were simply because I weighed too much. One of these was to take a ride in a hot-air balloon, something that I have wanted to do ever since I saw several in the air above me on the summer day in 2004 when I arrived in Boulder, Colorado, where I now live. I checked it out and found that they have an individual weight limit of 250 pounds. Now that I am well below that limit, I'm going for one of those rides. In fact, that will be the way that I will mark my dual celebration of my success in getting down to a normal weight and having this book published.

Now it's your time to think how you will celebrate your weight-loss success. The next step after setting your goal is to decide how you want to celebrate when you reach it. It doesn't have to be a hot-air balloon ride or a meal at a fancy restaurant—which might be too big for you to enjoy anyway. Maybe the best celebration is something you just couldn't do before you reached your goal. How are you going to celebrate when you reach your goal weight?

Endnotes

INTRODUCTION

xxv   *Nurses' Health Study:* Eunyoung Cho et al., "A Prospective Study of Obesity and Risk of Coronary Heart Disease Among Diabetic Women," *Diabetes Care,* 25:1142–1148 (July 2002).

1. DIABETES AND WEIGHT: WHY DIABETES DOESN'T MAKE YOU FAT

1   *almost exactly two-thirds:* The National Institute of Diabetes and Digestive and Kidney Diseases (NIDDK) of the National Institutes of Health (NIH), "Statistics Related to Overweight and Obesity," October 2006, win.niddk.nih.gov/statistics/index.htm (12 December 2006).

1   *body mass index:* Centers for Disease Control and Prevention, "BMI—Body Mass Index: About BMI for Adults," 30 May 2006, www.cdc.gov/nccdphp/dnpa/bmi/adult_BMI/about_adult_BMI.htm (12 December 2006).

2   *7 percent of us have diabetes:* National Center for Chronic Disease Prevention and Health Promotion of the Centers for Disease Control and Prevention, "National Diabetes Fact Sheet 2005," 16 November 2006, www.cdc.gov/diabetes/pubs/estimates05.htm (12 December 2006).

2   *one-fourth of Americans with prediabetes:* The National Institute of Diabetes and Digestive and Kidney Diseases (NIDDK) of the National Institutes of Health (NIH),

"National Diabetes Statistics," November 2005,
diabetes.niddk.nih.gov/dm/pubs/statistics/ (12 December
2006) for "at least 54 million American adults had prediabetes
in 2002." U.S. Census Bureau, "national population
estimates—characteristics," 6 August 2004,
www.census.gov/popest/archives/2000s/vintage_2002/
NA-EST2002-ASRO–01.html (12 December 2006) for total
population of 288,368,698 less 81,022,584 under 20 years
equals 207,346,114 or 26 percent with prediabetes in 2002.

2   *more than 85 percent of people with diabetes are overweight
or obese:* Centers for Disease Control and Prevention,
"Prevalence of Overweight and Obesity among Adults with
Diagnosed Diabetes—United States, 1988–1994 and
1999–2002," *Morbidity and Mortality Weekly Report,* 18
November 2004, www.cdc.gov/MMWR/preview/mmwrhtml/
mm5345a2.htm (12 December 2006).

3   *obesity causes about two-thirds of diabetes:* Cited in J. Eric
Oliver, *Fat Politics: The Real Story behind America's Obesity
Epidemic* (New York: Oxford University Press, 2006), pp. 49–50.

3   *"Daniel Porte Jr.:"* Author's interview with Dr. Porte, 8
September 2000.

2. OUR DOUBLE BIND: WHICH DIABETES DRUGS LEAD TO GAINING WEIGHT

7   *Only 15 percent:* National Center for Chronic Disease
Prevention and Health Promotion of the Centers for Disease
Control and Prevention, "Insulin and Diabetes Medication
Use," *National Diabetes Surveillance System,* 27 May 2005,
www.cdc.gov/diabetes/statistics/meduse/fig3.htm
(13 December 2006).

7   *Banting and Best:* Michael Bliss, *The Discovery of Insulin*
(Toronto: McClelland and Stewart, 1982).

8   *UKPDS:* "United Kingdom Prospective Diabetes Study 24:
A 6-Year, Randomized, Controlled Trial Comparing

Sulfonylurea, Insulin, and Metformin Therapy in Patients with Newly Diagnosed Type 2 Diabetes That Could Not Be Controlled with Diet Therapy," *Annals of Internal Medicine,* 128:165–175 (1 February 1998).

8   *Comi:* Richard Comi, "Treatment of Type 2 Diabetes Mellitus: A Weighty Enigma," *Annals of Internal Medicine,* 143:609–610 (18 October 2005).

9   *about a dozen brands of sulfonylureas:* David Mendosa, "Part 11: Diabetes Medications Web Sites," *On-line Diabetes Resources,* 11 December 2006, www.mendosa.com/ drugs.htm (18 December 2006).

10   *Kaiser:* Gregory A. Nichols and Andres Gomez, "Weight Changes Associated with Anti-Hyperglycemic Therapies for Type 2 Diabetes," Abstract 13-OR, 66th Annual Scientific Sessions of the American Diabetes Association, San Diego, 10–14 June 2005.

10   *Glucophage:* Bristol-Myers Squibb Company, "GLUCOPHAGE® (metformin hydrochloride tablets)" [prescribing information], March 2004, www.glucophagexr.com/cgi-bin/anybin.pl?sql =select%20PPI%20from%20TB_PRODUCT_PPI%20 where%20PPI_SEQ=52&key=PPI (18 December 2006).

11   *Precose (acarbose):* Bayer Pharmaceuticals Corporation, "PRECOSE® (acarbose tablets)" [prescribing information], November 2004, www.univgraph.com/Bayer/inserts/ Precose.pdf (18 December 2006).

11   *Glyset (miglitol):* Pharmacia and Upjohn Company, "Glyset (miglitol) Tablet, Film Coated" [prescribing information], March 2006, dailymed.nlm.nih.gov/dailymed/ drugInfo.cfm?id=503 (18 December 2006).

11   *Avandia (rosiglitazone):* GlaxoSmithKline, "Prescribing Information: Avandia® (rosiglitazone maleate) Tablets," September 2006, us.gsk.com/products/assets/us_avandia.pdf (18 December 2006).

11   *Actos (pioglitazone):* Takeda Pharmaceuticals America, Inc., "ACTOS® (pioglitazone hydrochloride) Tablets," November 2006, www.actos.com/pi.pdf (18 December 2006).

12   *Prandin (repaglinide):* Novo Nordisk A/S, "PRANDIN® (repaglinide) Tablets," 19 June 2006, www.prandin.com/docs/prandin_insert.pdf (18 December 2006).

12   *Starlix (nateglinide):* Novartis Pharmaceuticals Corporation, "Starlix® (nateglinide) tablets," November 2006, www.pharma.us.novartis.com/product/pi/pdf/Starlix.pdf (18 December 2006).

12   *Symlin (pramlintide):* Amylin Pharmaceuticals, Inc., "SYMLIN® (Pramlintide Acetate) Injection," June 2005, www.symlin.com/PDF/HCP/SYMLIN-pi-combined.pdf (18 December 2006).

13   *Byetta (exenatide):* Amylin Pharmaceuticals, Inc., "BYETTA® Exenatide Injection," October 2006, pi.lilly.com/us/byetta-pi.pdf (18 December 2006).

14   *Januvia (sitagliptin):* Merck & Co., Inc., "Highlights of Prescribing Information," October 2006, www.merck.com/product/usa/pi_circulars/j/januvia/januvia_pi.pdf (18 December 2006).

3. Byetta's Cousins: Other GLP-1 Mimetics in Development

18   *don't cover lunch:* Bernard Zinman et al., "Safety and Efficacy of Exenatide in Patients with Type 2 Diabetes Mellitus Using Thiazolidenediones with or without Metformin," Abstract 117-OR, 66th Annual Scientific Sessions of the American Diabetes Association, Washington, D.C., 10 June 2006, scientificsessions.diabetes.org/index.cfm?fuseaction=Locator.SearchAbstracts&CalledByID=1006 (21 December 2006).

18   *exenatide LAR:* Amylin Pharmaceuticals, Inc., "Form 10-Q Quarterly Report," 7 August 2006, library.corporate-ir.net/

library/10/101/101911/items/208861/2006_2Q.pdf
(21 December 2006).

18   *posters:* Dennis Kim et al., "Safety and Effects of a Once-
Weekly, Long-Acting Release Formulation of Exenatide over
15 Weeks in Patients with Type 2 Diabetes," Abstract 487-P,
66th Annual Scientific Sessions of the American Diabetes
Association, Washington, D.C., 11 June 2006,
scientificsessions.diabetes.org/index.cfm?fuseaction=Locator
.SearchAbstracts&CalledByID=1006 (21 December 2006).

18   *leptin:* Amylin Pharmaceuticals, Inc., "Late Breaking Data
at ADA 2006 Shows Amylin-Leptin Co-Administration
Reduces Body Weight and Body Fat in Animal Studies," 10
June 2006, investors.amylin.com/phoenix.zhtml
?c=101911&p=irol-newsArticle_Print&ID=871151
&highligh= (27 December 2006); Jonathan Roth et al.,
"Leptin Responsivity Restored in Leptin-Resistant Diet-
Induced Obese (DIO) Rats: Synergistic Actions of Amylin
and Leptin for Reduction in Body Weight (BW) and Fat,"
Abstract 52-LB, 66th Annual Scientific Sessions of the
American Diabetes Association, Washington, D.C., 12 June
2006, scientificsessions.diabetes.org/index.cfm?fuseaction
=Locator.SearchAbstracts&CalledByID=1006 (27
December 2006); and Kelly Close, *Diabetes Close Up,*
December 2006, closeconcerns.com/dcu-issue.php?issue=64
(27 December 2006).

19   *Liraglutide:* Novo Nordisk A/S, "Liraglutide (NN2211),"
n.d., www.novonordisk.com/press/rd_pipeline/rd_pipeline
.asp?showid=4 (21 December 2006).

19   *launch it in 2009:* Kelly Close, *Diabetes Close Up,*
November 2006, www.closeconcerns.com/dcu-back-
issues.php#2006 (21 December 2006).

20   *one clinical trial:* Tina Vilsboll et al., "Liraglutide
Significantly Improves Glycemic Control, and Lowers Body
Weight without Risk of Either Major or Minor

Hypoglycemic Episodes in Subjects with Type 2 Diabetes," Abstract 115-OR, 66th Annual Scientific Sessions of the American Diabetes Association, Washington, D.C., 10 June 2006, scientificsessions.diabetes.org/index.cfm?fuseaction =Locator.SearchAbstracts&CalledByID=1006 (21 December 2006).

20   *renders it resistant:* J.F. Todd and S.R. Bloom, "**Incretins** and Other Peptides in the Treatment of Diabetes," *Diabetic Medicine,* 24:223–232 (March 2007).

21   *monkeys they tested:* Laurie L. Baggio et al., "The Long-Acting Albumin-Exendin-4 GLP-1R Agonist CJC-1134 Engages Central and Peripheral Mechanisms Regulating Glucose Homeostasis," Abstract 362-OR, 66th Annual Scientific Sessions of the American Diabetes Association, Washington, D.C., 13 June 2006, scientificsessions.diabetes .org/index.cfm?fuseaction=Locator.SearchAbstracts&Called ByID=1006 (21 December 2006), and Karen Thibaudeau et al., "CJC-1134-PC: An Exendin-4 Conjugate with Extended Pharmacodynamic Profiles in Rodents," Abstract 434-P, 66th Annual Scientific Sessions of the American Diabetes Association, Washington, D.C., 12 June 2006, scientificsessions.diabetes.org/index.cfm?fuseaction=Locator .SearchAbstracts&CalledByID=1006 (21 December 2006).

21   *press release:* ConjuChem Biotechnologies Inc., "Conjuchem's PC-DAC™: Exendin-4 Presented at the American Diabetes Association Annual Meeting," 13 June 2006, conjuchem.hyphenhealth.com/news/ ADA%20EN%20PR%20June%2013.pdf (21 December 2006).

21   *bad news:* ConjuChem Biotechnologies Inc., "PC-DAC™: Exendin-4 Phase I/II Multiple-Dose Study Preliminary Results Demonstrate Safety and Efficacy at Once-Weekly Dosing," 27 March 2007, conjuchem.hyphenhealth.com/ news/PR_EN_Results_March_26.pdf (20 May 2007).

21   *GSK716155 (formerly Albugon):* Human Genome Sciences
      Inc., "Human Genome Sciences Announces Financial
      Results for 2006 and Progress toward Commercialization,"
      27 February 2006, www.hgsi.com/news/press/07-02-27_4
      Qtr&FY_2006_Results.htm (8 March 2007); Laurie L.
      Baggio et al., "A Recombinant Human Glucagon-Like
      Peptide (GLP)-1-Albumin Protein (Albugon) Mimics
      Peptidergic Activation of GLP-1 Receptor–Dependent
      Pathways Coupled with Satiety, Gastrointestinal Motility,
      and Glucose Homeostasis," *Diabetes:* 53:2492–2500
      (September 2004).

21   *LY 548806:* Kimberley Jackson et al., "Pharmacodynamic
      and Pharmacokinetic Properties of LY 548806, a GLP-1
      Analogue Optimized for IV Use," Abstract 562-P, 66th
      Annual Scientific Sessions of the American Diabetes
      Association, Washington, D.C., 10–14 June 2006,
      scientificsessions.diabetes.org/Abstracts/index.cfm?fuseaction
      =Locator.SearchAbstracts (21 December 2006).

22   *BIM51077:* Christoph Kapitza et al., "BIM51077, a Novel
      GLP-1 Analog, Achieves Sustained Improvement in Blood
      Glucose Control over 28 Days of Treatment," Abstract 500-
      P, 66th Annual Scientific Sessions of the American Diabetes
      Association, Washington, D.C., 11 June 2006,
      scientificsessions.diabetes.org/index.cfm?fuseaction=Locator
      .SearchAbstracts&CalledByID=1006 (21 December 2006);
      Joaquin Ramis et al., "Pharmacokinetic Profile of a SRF
      Formulation of BIM51077, a Novel GLP-1 Analog, in the
      Beagle Dog," Abstract 547-P, 66th Annual Scientific
      Sessions of the American Diabetes Association, Washington,
      D.C., 11 June 2006, scientificsessions.diabetes.org/index.cfm
      ?fuseaction=Locator.SearchAbstracts&CalledByID=1006
      (21 December 2006); and Christoph Kapitza et al.,
      "BIM51077, a Novel GLP-1 Analog, Showed Linear PK and

Dose-Response Relationship over 7 Days of Treatment,"
Abstract 2019-PO, 66th Annual Scientific Sessions of the
American Diabetes Association, Washington, D.C., June
2006, scientificsessions.diabetes.org/index.cfm?fuseaction
=Locator.SearchAbstracts&CalledByID=1006
(21 December 2006).

22   *Ipsen:* Ipsen, "Type 2 Diabetes Therapy: Ipsen is Currently
Testing an Innovative Sustained Release Formulation of its
GLP-1 Analogue Based on Its Proprietary Drug Delivery
System Technologies," 12 June 2006, investors.ipsen.com/
fichiers/fckeditor/File/PR_ADA&BIM51077_EN.pdf
(21 December 2006).

22   *phase 2b:* Sanofi-Aventis, "Metabolic Disorders," *R&D
Portfolio*, 7 November 2006, http://en.sanofi-aventis.com/
rd/portfolio/p_rd_portfolio_metabo.asp
(21 December 2006).

22   *BioRexis:* Jie Zhou et al., "Glucagon-like Peptide-1/Human
Transferrin Fusion Protein is a Potent Anti-hypergenic Agent"
[poster presented at the June 2005 meeting of the Endocrine
Society], www.biorexis.com/content/productPipeline/
documents/ENDOPosterJune2005.pdf (18 February 2007).

22   *clinical trial process:* Zeke Ashton, "Clinical Trials and the
FDA," *The Motley Fool*, 5 April 2000, www.fool.com/Server/
printarticle.aspx?file=/specials/2000/sp000405fda.htm
(21 December 2006).

4. OTHER TYPES OF WEIGHT-LOSS DRUGS

25   *Xenical:* Roche Laboratories Inc, "Xenical® (orlistat)
Capsules," January 2005, www.rocheusa.com/products/
xenical/pi.pdf (9 January 2007).

26   *Meridia:* Abbott Laboratories, "Meridia® (sibutramine
hydrochloride monohydrate) Capsules," August 2006,
www.rxabbott.com/pdf/meridia.pdf (24 December 2006)
and ME Lean, "Sibutramine—A Review of Clinical

Efficacy," *International Journal of Obesity and Related Metabolic Disorders*, 1997 Mar; 21 Suppl 1:S30–36.

26   *Alli:* U.S. Food and Drug Administration, "FDA Approves Orlistat for Over-the-Counter Use," 7 February 2007, www.fda.gov/bbs/topics/NEWS/2007/NEW01557.html (9 February 2007).

27   *over-the-counter drugs to lose weight:* Marilynn Larkin, "Ways to Win at Weight Loss," *FDA Consumer,* revised May 1999.

28   *CLA:* Leah D. Whigham et al., "Efficacy of Conjugated Linoleic Acid for Reducing Fat Mass: A Meta-analysis in Humans," *American Journal of Clinical Nutrition,* 85:1203–1211 (May 2007).

28   *Hoodia:* Jasjit S. Bindra, "A Popular Pill's Hidden Danger," *New York Times,* 26 April 2005, query.nytimes.com/gst/fullpage.html?res=9505E3D71231F935A15757C0A9639C8B63 (December 28, 2006).

29   *CP-945,598:* Pfizer, "Capitalizing on Expanded Opportunities: Cardiovascular, Metabolic, and Endocrine Disease (CVMED)," 30 November 2006, media.pfizer.com/pfizer/download/investors/presentations/Ryder_112906_part1.pdf (27 December 2006).

29   *Adyvia:* Innodia, "Adyvia™," 2006, http://www.innodia-inc.com/en/product-pipeline/adyvia.php (26 December 2006).

29   *CP404:* Compellis Pharmaceuticals, Inc., "Compellis Pharmaceuticals Awarded Patent for Its Therapeutic Platform for Treating Obesity," 5 December 2006, www.compellis.com/Press_release_Dec_06_copy(1).htm (26 December 2006).

30   *Excalia:* Orexigen Therapeutics, Inc., "Orexigen™ Therapeutics Reports Positive Phase II Results for Excalia™ Combination-Therapy to Treat Obesity," 22 October 2006, www.orexigen.com/news/news.php?id=10 (27 December 2006).

30   *oleoyl-estrone:* Manhattan Pharmaceuticals Inc., "Oleoyl-estrone" 10 May 2007, www.manhattanpharma.com/ (20 May 2007).

5. Back When Byetta Began: Why a Poisonous Lizard Is Good for You

32   *Dr. Eng:* Largely based on author's interviews with Dr. Eng, 16 April 2002 and 4 October 2006.

34   *his initial findings:* John Eng et al., "Purification and Structure of Exendin-3, A New Pancreatic Secretagogue Isolated from *Heloderma horridum* Venom," *Journal of Biological Chemistry*, 265:20259–20262 (25 November 1990).

34   *first article on exendin:* John Eng et al., "Isolation and Characterization of Exendin-4, an Exendin-3 Analogue, from *Heloderma suspectum* Venom," *Journal of Biological Chemistry*, 267:7402–7405 (15 April 1992).

35   *Exendin-4 required patent protection:* Kelly Close, "The Excitement Called Byetta and the Inspiration of Dr. John Eng," *Diabetes Close Up*, April 2005, www.closeconcerns .com/dcu-issue.php?issue=47 (28 December 2006).

35   *patent 5,424,286:* United States Patent 5,424,286, "Exendin-3 and Exendin-4 Polypeptides, and Pharmaceutical Compositions Comprising Same," *USPTO Patent Full-Text and Image Database*, 13 June 1995, patft.uspto.gov/netacgi/ nph-Parser?Sect2=PTO1&Sect2=HITOFF&p=1&u=%2 Fnetahtml%2Fsearch-bool.html&r=1&f=G&l=50&d =PALL&RefSrch=yes&Query=PN%2F5424286 (29 December 2006).

6. Byetta's Spectacular Launch

37   *aspirin:* Mary Bellis, History of Aspirin, "About: Inventors," 2006, inventors.about.com/library/inventors/blaspirin.htm (2 January 2007).

40   *Presentations:* 66th Scientific Sessions of the American Diabetes Association, Washington, D.C., June 2006, scientificsessions.diabetes.org/index.cfm?fuseaction=Locator. DisplaySearchAbstract&CalledByID=1006 (5 January 2007).

40   *Alex Berenson:* Alex Berenson, "A Ray of Hope for Diabetics,"
      New York Times, 2 March 2006, www.nytimes.com/
      2006/03/02/business/02drug.html?ex=1298955600&en=bdf9
      2ce6e341d57d&ei=5088 (5 January 2007).

7. How GLP-1 Mimetics Work

43   *they work in so many ways:* Daniel J. Drucker and Michael A.
      Nauck, "The Incretin System: Glucagon-like Peptide-1
      Receptor Agonists and Dipeptidyl Peptidase-4 Inhibitors in Type
      2 Diabetes," *Lancet,* 368:1696–1705 (11 November 2006).
45   *hypothalamus:* Kathleen Dungan and John B. Buse,
      "Glucagon-like Peptide-1–Based Therapies for Type 2
      Diabetes: A Focus on Exenatide," *Clinical Diabetes,*
      23:56–62 (April 2005).
48   *Monnier:* Louis Monnier, Hélène Lapinski, and Claude
      Colette, "Contributions of Fasting and Postprandial
      Plasma Glucose Increments to the Overall Diurnal
      Hyperglycemia of Type 2 Diabetic Patients: Variations
      with increasing levels of HbA$_{1c}$, *Diabetes Care,*
      26:881–885 (March 2003).

8. Can You Use Byetta? The Diabetes Advantage

54   *Gastroparesis:* Gastroparesis Clinical Research Consortium,
      "Request for Applications (RFA) Number: RFA-DK-05-004,"
      grants.nih.gov/grants/guide/rfa-files/RFA-DK-05-004.html
      (14 January 2007).
55   *Wyoming:* State of Wyoming (1 June 2004), "Wyoming
      Clinical Practice Recommendations for Diabetes Mellitus,"
      wdh.state.wy.us/DIABETES/pdf/dmcpr.pdf (16 January 2007).
55   *National Center:* National Center for Chronic Disease
      Prevention and Health Promotion, "Frequently Asked
      Questions," 27 June 2006, www.cdc.gov/DIABETES/faq/
      concerns.htm (16 January 2007). See also: National Digestive
      Diseases Information Clearinghouse, "Gastroparesis and

Diabetes," December 2003, digestive.niddk.nih.gov/ddiseases/
pubs/gastroparesis/index.htm (22 January 2007).

55 *our genes:* Martin Beinborn et al., "A Human Glucagon-like
Peptide-1 Receptor Polymorphism Results in Reduced Agonist
Responsiveness," *Regulatory Peptides,* 130:1–6 (15 August 2005).

9. Problems with Byetta

61 *77 degrees F:* Amylin Pharmaceuticals Inc., "Patient Information,"
February 2007, pi.lilly.com/us/byetta-ppi.pdf (16 February 2007).

10. When Byetta Fails

69 *most influential article:* Alex Berenson, "A Ray of Hope for
Diabetics," *New York Times,* 2 March 2006,
www.nytimes.com/2006/03/02/business/02drug.html?ex=1298
955600&en=bdf92ce6e341d57d&ei=5088 (23 January 2007).

72 *Dr. Joe:* "J. Joseph Prendergast, M.D.," 15 October 2006,
www.endocrinemetabolic.com/about/jjp.htm (23 January 2007).

73 *Diabetes for Dummies:* "DrRubin.com," www.mendosa.com/
subscribe.htm (23 January 2007).

73 *Diabetes Update:* You can subscribe to my free online newsletter,
"Diabetes Update," at www.mendosa.com/subscribe.htm.

73 *diabetes podcasts:* David Mendosa, "Diabetes Podcasts, 14
September 2006, www.healthcentral.com/diabetes/
c/17/2295/diabetes-podcasts/pf/ (23 January 2007).

74 *Weight, Weight Don't Tell Me!:* http://wtwt.endocrinemetabolic
.com/ (23 January 2007).

11. The GLP-1 Lifestyle

76 *Byetta Web site:* "Efficacy," 2006, www.byetta.com/hcp/
byetta_efficacy_222.jsp?reqNavId=2.3 (29 January 2007).

76 *Rethinking Thin:* Gina Kolata, *Rethinking Thin: The New
Science of Weight Loss—and the Myths and Realities of
Dieting* (New York: Farrar, Straus and Giroux, 2007).

78   *Roy Walford and his daughter Lisa:* Roy L. Walford, *Beyond the 120 Year Diet: How to Double Your Vital Years,* revised edition (New York: Four Walls Eight Windows, 2000); Brian M. Delaney and Lisa Walford, *The Longevity Diet: Discover Calorie Restriction—The Only Proven Way to Slow the Aging Process and Maintain Peak Vitality* (New York: Marlowe & Company, 2005).

78   *long, miserable life:* Rebecca Traister, "Diet Your Way to a Long, Miserable Life! 'Calorie Restricted' Eaters Have Visions of Eternal Health Dancing in Their Heads. But Is Life without Pecan Pie Really Worth Living?" *Salon,* 22 November 2006, www.salon.com/mwt/feature/2006/11/22/cr_diets/print.html (11 February 2007).

79   *homocysteine:* David Mendosa, "Homocysteine," 21 August 2002, www.mendosa.com/homocysteine.htm (11 February 2007).

79   *magnesium:* David Mendosa, "Magnesium and Diabetes," 24 May 2006, www.healthcentral.com/diabetes/c/17/1672/magnesium-diabetes/pf/ (11 February 2007).

79   *vitamin D:* John N. Hathcock et al., "Risk Assessment for Vitamin D," *American Journal of Clinical Nutrition,* 85:6–18 (January 2007).

79   *Steven Bratman:* David Mendosa, "Alternative Therapies for Diabetes," 29 November 2006, www.mendosa.com/alternative_therapies.htm (11 February 2007).

80   *protein:* Food and Nutrition Board, Institute of Medicine, *Dietary Reference Intakes for Energy, Carbohydrate, Fiber, Fat, Fatty Acids, Cholesterol, Protein, and Amino Acids (Macronutrients)* (Washington, D.C.: National Academy of Sciences, 2005), p. 645.

12. THE GLYCEMIC AND SATIETY INDEXES

84   *You can benefit from eating low glycemic:* Joanna McMillan-Price and Jennie Brand-Miller, "Low-Glycaemic Index

Diets and Body Weight Regulation," *International Journal of Obesity*, 30:S40–S46 (December 2006).

84 *metabolic rate:* Babak Bahadori et al., "Low-Fat, High-Carbohydrate (Low-Glycaemic Index) Diet Induces Weight Loss and Preserves Lean Body Mass in Obese Healthy Subjects: Results of a 24-Week Study," *Diabetes, Obesity and Metabolism*, 7:290–293 (May 2005).

89 *satiety index:* David Mendosa, "What Really Satisfies," *Diabetes Interview*, May 1998; you can also find this article on my Web site at www.mendosa.com/satiety.htm.

13. SPICE UP YOUR LIFE

92 *metabolic effect:* Margriet Westerterp-Plantenga et al., "Metabolic Effects of Spices, Teas, and Caffeine," *Physiology & Behavior*, 89:85–91 (30 August 2006).

93 *Penzeys Spices:* This Brookfield, Wisconsin, company does most of its business by mail order and on the Web at penzeys.com. But it also has more than 30 stores, including a new one near me in Arvada, Colorado, where I can see and sniff the spices before buying.

93 *Upton Tea Imports:* This Hopkinton, Massachusetts, company does most of its business by mail order and on the Web at uptontea.com. Its teas are first-rate, its people are knowledgeable, and their service is great.

14. DAVID'S DIABETES DIET

95 *new nutrition recommendations:* American Diabetes Association, "Nutrition Recommendations and Interventions for Diabetes—2006: A position statement of the American Diabetes Association," *Diabetes Care*, 20:2140–2157 (September 2006).

97 *chana dal:* David Mendosa, "Chana Dal," 11 November 2006, www.mendosa.com/chanadal.html (19 February 2007).

98   *UC Berkeley Wellness Letter:* University of California,
     Berkeley, Wellness Letter, Subscription Department, P.O.
     Box 420148, Palm Coast, FL 32142; toll-free telephone
     800-829-9170.

98   *people who eat salads:* L. Joseph Su and Lenore Arab, "Salad
     and Raw Vegetable Consumption and Nutritional Status in the
     Adult US Population: Results from the Third National Health
     and Nutrition Examination Survey," *Journal of the American
     Dietetic Association,* 106:1394–1404 (September 2006).

99   *National Barley Foods Council:* National Barley Foods Council,
     "BarleyFoods," www.barleyfoods.org/ (20 February 2007).

99   *dietary guidelines:* U.S. Department of Health and Human
     Services and the U.S. Department of Agriculture, "Dietary
     Guidelines for Americans 2005," 25 May 2005,
     www.health.gov/dietaryguidelines/dga2005/document/
     (20 February 2007).

99   *Bob's Red Mill:* Bob's Red Mill Natural Foods, 5209 SE
     International Way, Milwaukie, OR 97222; toll-free
     800-349-2173; bobsredmill.com.

101 *Golden Barley Cereal:* Whole Control LLC, 6360 Quail
     Street, Arvada, CO 80004; toll-free 888-946-5326;
     whole-control.com.

101 *Fats That Heal, Fats That Kill:* Udo Erasmus, *Fats That
     Heal, Fats That Kill: The Complete Guide to Fats, Oils,
     Cholesterol and Human Health,* revised edition (Burnaby,
     BC, Canada: Alive Books, 1993).

102 *fiber:* Denis Lairon et al., "Dietary Fiber Intake and Risk
     Factors for Cardiovascular Disease in French Adults,"
     American Journal of Clinical Nutrition, 82:1185–1194
     (December 2005).

105 *Weil:* Andrew Weil, "Aspartame: Can a Little Bit Hurt?" 9
     May 2006, www.drweil.com/drw/u/id/QAA106654
     (22 February 2007).

106   *two dozen patent applications:* U.S. Patent & Trademark
       Office, appft1.uspto.gov/netacgi/nph-Parser?Sect1
       =PTO2&Sect2=HITOFF&u=%2Fnetahtml%2FPTO%2Fs
       earch-adv.html&r=0&p=1&f=S&l=50&Query=an%2Fcoca-
       cola+and+stevia&d=PG01 (31 May 2007).

108   *organic foods:* Danny K. Asami et al., "Comparison of the
       Total Phenolic and Ascorbic Acid Content of Freeze-Dried
       and Air-Dried Marionberry, Strawberry, and Corn Grown
       Using Conventional, Organic, and Sustainable
       Agricultural Practices," *Journal of Agricultural and Food
       Chemistry,* 51:1237–1241 (26 February 2003); Donald R.
       Davis et al., "Changes in USDA Food Composition Data
       for 43 Garden Crops, 1950 to 1999," *Journal of the
       American College of Nutrition,* 23:669–682 (December
       2004).

16. Sugars

113   *sugar:* American Diabetes Association, "Sugar & Sugar
       Substitutes," www.diabetes.org/for-parents-and-kids/diabetes-
       care/sugar.jsp (22 February 2007).

114   *molasses:* Ruth H. Matthews, Palema R. Pehrsson, and
       Mojgan Farhat-Sabet, "Sugar Content of Selected Foods:
       Individual and Total Sugars," Home Economics Research
       Report No. 48, Human Nutrition Information Service, U.S.
       Department of Agriculture, September 1987,
       www.nal.usda.gov/fnic/foodcomp/Data/Other/herr48.pdf
       (23 February 2007).

114   *rotting teeth:* Paula J. Moynihan and Poul Erik Petersen,
       "Diet, Nutrition and the Prevention of Dental Diseases,"
       Public Health Nutrition, 7:201–226 (February 2004).

114–   *many people link:* Sharon S. Elliott et al, "Fructose, weight
115   gain, and the insulin resistance syndrome," *American
       Journal of Clinical Nutrition,* 76:911–922 (November 2002).

115 *some people:* Joe Anderson, "AGEs and Aging-Sweet Suicide," 9 November 2006, andersonclan.us/andersonclan_top/ages.html (23 February 2007).

116 *the ADA says:* American Diabetes Association, "Evidence-Based Nutrition Principles and Recommendations for the Treatment and Prevention of Diabetes and Related Complications: Position Statement," *Diabetes Care,* 25:202–212 (January 2002).

116 *pros and cons of using fructose:* John P. Bantle, "Is Fructose the Optimal Low Glycemic Index Sweetener?" *Nestlé Nutrition Workshop Series: Clinical & Performance Programme,* 11:83–91 (2006).

116 *earlier research:* John P. Bantle et al., "Effects of Dietary Fructose on Plasma Lipids in Healthy Subjects," *American Journal of Clinical Nutrition,* 72: 1128–1134 (November 2000).

17. BAD FATS

119 *Dietary cholesterol:* D. Kritchevsky, "Diet and Atherosclerosis," *Journal of Nutrition, Health and Aging,* 5:155–159 (2001).

119 *association of cholesterol, saturated fat:* J. Michael Gaziano and JoAnn E. Manson, "Diet and Heart Disease. The Role of Fat, Alcohol, and Antioxidants," *Cardiology Clinics,* 14:69–83 (February 1996).

120 *Saturated fat reduction is a primary goal:* Amy E. Griel and Penny M. Kris-Etherton, "Beyond Saturated Fat: The Importance of the Dietary Fatty Acid Profile on Cardio-vascular Disease." *Nutrition Reviews,* 64: 257–262 (May 2006).

120 *another medical researcher:* Günther Wolfram, "Dietary Fatty Acids and Coronary Heart Disease," *European Journal of Medical Research,* 8:321–324 (20 August 2003).

120 *its proportion of saturated and unsaturated fat:* DietaryFiberFood.com "Fat: Total and Saturated Fat

Content in Food," 2006, www.dietaryfiberfood.com/fat-saturated.php (8 March 2007).

120   *Dr. Atkins:* Robert C. Atkins, *Dr. Atkins' New Diet Revolution,* revised edition (New York: M. Evans, 2003).

120   *cream has more saturated fat:* DietaryFiberFood.com, "Fat: Total and Saturated Fat Content in Cheese, Cream, Egg, and Milk and Their Products," 2006, www.dietaryfiberfood .com/fat-saturated2.php (8 March 2007).

121   *Spectrum Spread:* Spectrum Organic Products, Inc. in Petaluma, California, makes this healthy butter substitute. Spectrum is now part of The Hain Celestial Group, headquartered in Melville, New York.

122   *Institute of Medicine:* Institute of Medicine, "Letter Report on Dietary Reference Intakes for Trans Fatty Acids," 2002, www.iom.edu/Object.File/Master/13/083/TransFattyAcids.pdf (4 March 2007).

122   *Centers for Disease Control and Prevention:* National Center for Chronic Disease Prevention and Health Promotion of the Centers for Disease Control and Prevention, "National Diabetes Fact Sheet," *National Estimates on Diabetes,* 31 January 2005, www.cdc.gov/diabetes/pubs/estimates.htm (7 March 2007).

123   *The American Journal of Clinical Nutrition:* Jorge Salmerón et al., "Dietary Fat Intake and Risk of Type 2 Diabetes in Women," *American Journal of Clinical Nutrition,* 73:1019–1026 (June 2001).

124   *The FDA said:* Food and Drug Administration, "Food Labeling: Trans Fatty Acids in Nutrition Labeling, Nutrient Content Claims, and Health Claims; Proposed Rule,"12 November 1999, vm.cfsan.fda.gov/~lrd/fr991117.html (20 February 2007).

18. TIPS FOR WEIGHT LOSS

125   *Eating Rate and Satiation:* Ana Andrade, Tara Minaker, Kathleen Melanson, "Eating Rate and Satiation," Oral

Abstract Presentation, 21 October 2006, Annual Scientific
Meeting of NAASO, The Obesity Society, Boston, MA,
www.naaso.org/annualmeeting06/final_program.pdf
(15 February 2006).

126   *Mindless Eating*: David Mendosa, "Mindless Eating,"
www.diabetes-connections.com, 24 August 2006,
www.healthcentral.com/diabetes/c/17/2161/mindless-eating/pf/
(15 February 2007).

127   *size matters*: David Mendosa, "Size Matters," www.diabetes-
connections.com, 28 July 2006, www.healthcentral.com/
diabetes/c/17/2040/size-matters/pf/ (15 February 2007).

128   *Ron Krauss*: Gina Kolata, *Rethinking Thin: The New Science
of Weight Loss—And The Myths and Realities of Dieting*
(New York: Farrar, Straus and Giroux, 2007), p. 104.

128   *Coheso:* "Personal Health Management Tools," Coheso Inc.,
www.coheso.com (15 February 2007).

130   *downsize:* Tara Parker-Pope, "Small Steps: Easy Resolutions
for Healthier Living in 2007," *Wall Street Journal,* 2 January
2007.

131   *eating breakfast:* David Mendosa, "Eating to Lose Weight,"
www.diabetes-connections.com, 5 July 2006,
www.healthcentral.com/diabetes/c/17/1866/
eating-lose-weight/pf/ (15 February 2007).

133   *National Weight Control Registry:* "The National Weight
Control Registry," www.nwcr.ws/ (15 February 2007).

133   *Mayo Clinic Health Letter:* Mayo Clinic Health Letter,
January 2007.

19. INEFFICIENCY IS NEAT

136   *Science:* J. A. Levine et al., "Interindividual Variation in
Posture Allocation: Possible Role in Human Obesity,"
Science, 307:584–586 (January 28, 2005).

136   *Denise Grady:* "The Fit Tend to Fidget, and Biology May Be
Why, a Study Says," *New York Times,* January 28, 2005.

20. AEROBIC EXERCISE

139   *Dr. Bernstein's Diabetes Solution:* Richard K. Bernstein, *Dr. Bernstein's Diabetes Solution: The Complete Guide to Achieving Normal Blood Sugars,* newly revised and updated edition (Boston: Little, Brown, 2007).

140   *Diabetes for Dummies:* Alan L. Rubin, *Diabetes for Dummies,* second edition (Hoboken, NJ: Wiley Publishing, 2004).

140   *meta-analysis:* D. E. Thomas, E. J. Elliott, and G. A. Naughton, "Exercise for Type 2 Diabetes Mellitus," *Cochrane Database of Systematic Reviews,* 19 July 2006, www.mrw.interscience.wiley.com/cochrane/clsysrev/articles/CD002968/frame.html (11 March 2007).

141   *position statement:* American Diabetes Association, "Physical Activity/Exercise and Diabetes," 2002, care.diabetesjournals.org/cgi/content/full/27/suppl_1/s58 (4 February 2007).

144   *a major study:* I-Min Lee et al., "Physical Activity and Coronary Heart Disease in Women: Is 'No Pain, No Gain' Passé?" *JAMA,* 285:1447–1454 (March 21, 2001).

145   *Surgeon General:* U.S. Department of Health and Human Services, *Physical Activity and Health: A Report of the Surgeon General* (Centers for Disease Control and Prevention, National Center for Chronic Disease Prevention and Health Promotion, Washington, D.C., U.S. Government Printing Office, 1996).

145   *the government's current recommendation: Dietary Guidelines for Americans 2005,* 11 January 2005, www.health.gov/dietaryguidelines/dga2005/recommendations.htm (4 February 2007).

146   *2004 study:* C. A. Slentz et al., "Effects of the Amount of Exercise on Body Weight, Body Composition, and Measures of Central Obesity: STRRIDE—A Randomized Controlled

Study," *Archives of Internal Medicine*, 164:31–39 (12 January 2004).

21. RESISTANCE IS USEFUL

148   *The Wall Street Journal*: Kristi Essick, "Weighty Issues," *Wall Street Journal*, February 3, 2007.

148   *High-resistance exercise*: American Diabetes Association, "Physical Activity/Exercise and Diabetes," 2002, care.diabetesjournals.org/cgi/content/full/27/suppl_1/s58 (4 February 2007).

149   *Resistance Training and Type 2 Diabetes*: Neil Eves and Ronald Plotnikoff, "Resistance Training and Type 2 Diabetes: Considerations for Implementation at the Population Level," *Diabetes Care*, 29:1933–1941 (August 2006).

149   *The largest published study*: Stefano Balducci et al., "Is a Long-Term Aerobic Plus Resistance Training Program Feasible for and Effective on Metabolic Profiles in Type 2 Diabetic Patients?" *Diabetes Care*, 27:841–842 (March 2004).

149   *meta-analysis in* Diabetes Care: Neil J. Snowling and Will G. Hopkins, "Effects of Different Modes of Exercise Training on Glucose Control and Risk Factors for Complications in Type 2 Diabetic Patients: A meta-analysis," *Diabetes Care*, 29:2518–2527 (November 2006).

151   *Only 12 percent did weight training*: Ronald C. Plotnikoff, "Physical Activity in the Management of Diabetes: Population-Based Perspectives and Strategies," *Canadian Journal of Diabetes*, 30:52–62 (March 2006).

152   *American College of Sports Medicine*: A. Albright et al., "American College of Sports Medicine Position Stand: Exercise and Type 2 Diabetes," *Medicine and Science in Sports and Exercise*, 32:1345–1360 (July 2000).

152   *a similar recommendation:* American Diabetes Association, "Standards of Medical Care in Diabetes—2007," October 2006, care.diabetesjournals.org/cgi/content/full/30/suppl_1/S4 (9 February 2007).

22. METABOLISM AND EXERCISE

153   *only 58 percent:* Elaine H. Morrato et al., "Physical Activity in U.S. Adults with Diabetes and at Risk for Developing Diabetes, 2003," *Diabetes Care,* 30:203–209 (February 2007).

154   *Three Rockefeller University physicians:* Rudolph L. Leibel, MD, Michael Rosenbaum, MD, and Jules Hirsch, MD, "Changes in Energy Expenditure Resulting from Altered Body Weight," *New England Journal of Medicine,* 332:621–628 (March 9, 1995).

154   *nonresting energy expenditure:* F. Xavier Pi-Sunyer, MD, "Weight Loss in Type 2 Diabetic Patients," *Diabetes Care,* 28:1526–1527 (June 2005).

155   *people who are successful:* Roland L.Weinsier et al., "Free-Living Activity Energy Expenditure in Women Successful and Unsuccessful at Maintaining a Normal Body Weight," *American Journal of Clinical Nutrition,* 75:499–504 (March 2002).

155   *a third thing:* Barry E. Levin, "The Drive to Regain is Mainly in the Brain," *American Journal of Physiology—Regulatory, Integrative and Comparative Physiology,* 287(6):R1297–1300 (December 2004).

Resources

DAVID MENDOSA'S WEB SITE
www.mendosa.com/diabetes

This is a directory of articles, columns, and Web pages by David Mendosa, a freelance journalist specializing in diabetes. The site includes about 1,000 of his articles, his monthly "Diabetes Update" newsletters, links to his blog, and his annotated directory to more than 1,400 Web sites about diabetes, which are described and linked in the 16 pages of his "On-line Diabetes Resources."

DAVID MENDOSA'S DIABETES ARTICLES AT HEALTH CENTRAL
www.healthcentral.com/diabetes/c/17

This is where David Mendosa writes two new articles about all aspects of diabetes every week.

ENDOCRINE METABOLIC MEDICAL CENTER
www.endocrinemetabolic.com

This is the clinic of Dr. John Joseph Prendergast in Palo Alto, California. It approaches patient care with principles of integrative medicine and a focus on disease prevention.

This site links to his first book, *The Uncommon Doctor: Dr. Joe's Rx for Managing Your Health.*

DISCUSSION GROUPS ABOUT BYETTA

Dr. Bill Quick's discussion forum for Byetta is the most active one. The address is:

diabetes.blog.com

Diabetes_And_Byetta is the most active Yahoo group about Byetta. The address is:

health.groups.yahoo.com/group/Diabetes_And_Byetta

FURTHER INFORMATION ABOUT BYETTA

You can find more information on Byetta on the Web site at byetta.com and by calling the Amylin Lilly Customer Support Center toll-free at 1-800-868-1190.

Glossary

A1C: This is the key test that measures a person's average blood glucose level over the past two to three months. Sometimes doctors call it hemoglobin A1C or glycosylated or glycated hemoglobin. Hemoglobin is the part of a red blood cell that carries oxygen to the cells and sometimes joins with the glucose in the bloodstream. The test indicates the percentage of hemoglobin that is "glycated," i.e., has a glucose molecule riding on its back. This is proportional to the amount of glucose in the blood. The higher the level of A1C, the greater the risk of developing diabetic complications. If you have diabetes, you need to have your doctor measure it two to four times a year, depending on your type and how well you control your diabetes. You should certainly aim to keep it under 7 percent, and probably even lower.

Aerobic exercise: This type of exercise uses large muscle groups, can be maintained continuously, and is rhythmic in nature. It overloads the heart and lungs and causes them to work harder than at rest, improving the body's use of oxygen.

Albumin: This is a type of protein that dissolves in water and readily coagulates. Albumin helps to regulate the distribution of water in our body.

Analog: An analog (British English spells it analogue) is an organic compound with a molecular structure closely similar to another, typically differing in one atom or group. By this definition, liraglutide is a GLP-1 analog, but Byetta is not, because it is only about 50 percent homologous (similar in structure) to GLP-1.

Avandia: Avandia (rosiglitazone) is an oral medication for people with type 2 diabetes. Its side effects include weight gain. It may also cause heart attacks.

Beta cells: These cells produce the hormone insulin. They are found grouped together in the Islets of Langerhans in the pancreas.

Blood glucose: This is the most common kind of sugar found in the blood and is the main source of energy for most of the body's organs and tissues and the only source of fuel for the brain. When the body's digestive organs process carbohydrates, the food ends up as glucose that passes through the walls of the intestine into the bloodstream to the liver and eventually into general circulation. From here the glucose enters individual cells or tissues throughout the body to be used for fuel and provide energy.

Blood glucose level: This is the amount of glucose in your bloodstream. If you haven't eaten in the past few hours (and you don't have diabetes), your blood glucose level will normally fall within the range of 70–110 mg/dl (3.9–6 mmol/L). If you eat, this will rise, but rarely above 180 mg/dl (10 mmol/L). The extent of the increase will vary depending on your glucose tolerance (your own physiological response) and the type of food you have just eaten.

BMI: The Body Mass Index, a measure of body weight relative to height.

Byetta: This is Amylin Pharmaceuticals' brand name of exenatide.

Carbohydrate: This is one of the three main nutrients in food. Foods that are rich in carbohydrate are cereals and cereal products, including bread, cookies, pasta, some vegetables—particularly potatoes, sweet potatoes, and sweet corn—most fruits, dairy products (except cheese), and sugar, honey, jam, and candy.

Dawn phenomenon: This is the early-morning (about 4 A.M. to 8 A.M.) rise in blood glucose level. All of us, whether we have diabetes or not, experience the dawn phenomenon to some degree.

DPP-4: This is short for dipeptidyl peptidase-4, which is a new class of diabetes medications that a team of Danish researchers discovered in 1995. DPP-4 inhibit the enzyme that inactivates GLP-1. Drugs belonging to this class include sitagliptin (Januvia).

Exenatide: This is the synthetic version of a peptide, exendin-4, that Dr. John Eng first isolated from the salivary secretions of the Gila monster in the 1990s. Exenatide has a structure similar to that of human GLP-1, but unlike human GLP-1 it is resistant to degradation.

Fiber: This is a form of carbohydrate that passes through the human digestive tract without being digested. Fiber contributes neither calories nor a rise in blood glucose levels.

Gila monster: This poisonous lizard can go for a long time without eating. When studied, it was found to produce a protein that helped to slow the emptying of its stomach so that it stayed full. This protein is very similar to one that humans make called glucagonlike peptide-1 (GLP-1). Researchers have now made a synthetic GLP-1, which the U.S. Food and Drug Administration approved in 2005 for the treatment of type 2 diabetes. It is called exenatide and marketed under the brand name Byetta.

GLP-1: This is the common abbreviation for glucagonlike peptide-1.

Glucagon: The pancreas produces this hormone that stimulates an increase in blood glucose levels, thus countering the action of insulin.

Glucagonlike peptide-1: Often abbreviated as GLP-1, this peptide increases insulin secretion from the pancreas in a glucose-dependent manner. Joel Francis Habener of Harvard Medical School and three colleagues in 1982 first described it in anglerfish (monkfish). Human GLP-1 only works for a few minutes until the dipeptidyl peptidase-4 enzyme (DPP-4) makes it stop working.

Glycemic index: This is the system for ranking foods according to their impact on blood glucose levels. Foods with a high glycemic value raise blood glucose quicker and higher. It provides a ranking of carbohydrate-containing foods, based on the food's effect on blood glucose compared with a standard reference food.

Homocysteine: This is a toxic waste product produced during cellular metabolism. High levels of it are a risk factor for coronary artery disease.

Hormones: These are proteins produced by organs of the body that trigger activity in other locations.

Incretins: These are hormones that causes an increase in the amount of insulin released when glucose levels are normal and particularly when they are elevated. They also slow the rate of absorption of nutrients into the bloodstream, may reduce food intake, and inhibit glucagon release. The incretin effect describes the enhanced insulin response from orally ingested glucose compared with intravenous glucose leading to identical postprandial plasma glucose levels. It is responsible for up to 60 percent of the postprandial insulin secretion, but people with type 2 diabetes experience less of an effect than other people do. Long-acting drugs, like Byetta and liraglutide, which mimic the action of human GLP-1, are incretin mimetics. Some experts prefer to call Byetta an agonist of GLP-1. But agonist reminds us too much of agony. These terms come from the same Greek root, and the echoes of agony certainly aren't appropriate for something as positive as these drugs.

Insulin: This is a hormone produced by the beta cells of the pancreas that helps glucose pass into the cells, where it is used to create energy for the body. The pancreas should automatically produce the right amount of insulin to move glucose into the cells. When the body cannot make enough insulin, it has to be taken by injection or through use of an insulin pump. Insulin is not only involved in regulating blood glucose levels, it plays a key part in determining whether we burn fat or carbohydrate to meet our energy needs—it switches muscle cells from fat burning to carb burning. For this reason, lowering insulin levels is one of the secrets to lifelong health.

Insulin resistance: This is the condition in which normal amounts of insulin are inadequate to produce a normal insulin response from fat, muscle, and liver cells. The pancreas tries to keep up with the demand for insulin by producing more of it. Eventually, the pancreas cannot keep up with the body's need for insulin, and excess glucose builds up in the bloodstream. Insulin resistance can lead to type 2 diabetes.

Metabolism: This is the term used to describe how the cells of the body chemically change the food you consume and make the protein, fats, and carbohydrates into forms of energy, or use them for growth and repair.

Meta-analysis: A meta-analysis pools the result of previous separate but related studies. It overcomes the problem of reduced statistical power in studies with small sample sizes.

Metformin: This is the most commonly prescribed oral medication to lower blood glucose of people with type 2 diabetes.

mg/dl: This stands for milligrams per deciliter—a unit of measure that shows the concentration of a substance in a specific amount of fluid. In the United States, blood glucose test results are reported as mg/dl. Other countries, including Canada, use millimoles per liter (mmol/L). To convert blood glucose levels to mg/dl from mmol/L, multiply mmol/L by 18. Example: 10 mmol/L times18 equals 180 mg/dl.

mmol/L: This stands for millimoles per liter—a unit of measure that shows the concentration of a substance in a specific amount of fluid. Most of the world, including Canada, reports blood glucose test results as mmol/L. In the United States, we use milligrams per deciliter (mg/dl). To convert blood glucose results to mmol/L from mg/dl, divide mg/dL by 18. Example: 180 mg/dl divided by18 equals 10 mmol/L.

Obesity: This means a person's body mass index (BMI) is greater than 30 kg/m². The risk of developing prediabetes, type 2 diabetes, heart disease, stroke, and arthritis is very high when someone is obese.

Overweight: This means a person's body mass index (BMI) is between 25 and 29.9 kg/m². The healthy weight range is 18.5 to 24.9 kg/m². The risk of developing prediabetes, type 2 diabetes, heart disease, and stroke starts to increase when a person is overweight.

Pancreas: This is a vital organ behind the stomach that secretes the digestive juices that help break down food during digestion; it also produces the hormones insulin and glucagon.

Peptide hormones: These proteins are simple molecules made up of only a few amino acids.

Posters: All abstracts submitted for a scientific meeting may selected as abstracts only or abstracts that are presented as posters, which are displayed by category at the meeting in a specific location (sometimes called "the Poster Hall"). For each category, presenters are expected to be at their posters for a scheduled session lasting an hour or two.

Placebo: This is an inactive substance or preparation used as a control in an experiment or test to determine the effectiveness of a medicine.

Prandin: Prandin (repanglinide) is an oral medication for people with type 2 diabetes. It stimulates insulin secretion from the beta cells of the pancreas.

Resistance training: This is training designed to increase the body's strength, power, and muscular endurance through resistance exercise. This anaerobic (without oxygen) training includes weight training, weight machine use, and resistance band workouts.

Satiety: This is the condition of being full or gratified beyond the point of satisfaction; surfeit; having little hunger or appetite.

Starlix: Starlix (nateglinide) is an oral medication for people with type 2 diabetes. It restores early insulin secretion.

Sulfonylureas: These are a class of oral medicine for type 2 diabetes that lowers blood glucose by helping the pancreas make more insulin and by helping the body better use the insulin it makes.

Acknowledgments

First, I must give thanks to my wife, Catherine Lee Nord. She gave me encouragement and advice on the basis of her all too extensive knowledge of type 2 diabetes—a half century of living with it. Catherine died of diabetes complications. She lived long enough to know that I had finished this book but not to see it published.

Special thanks to Matthew Lore, who had the faith in me to publish this book. Matthew tried for years to have me write my own book for Marlowe & Company, and I finally found a subject that I knew well enough and had the passion to write about.

I am especially fortunate to have Gretchen Becker as a friend. Gretchen is the rare combination of a person who knows both what diabetes is and how to write about it. Her advice has been invaluable.

Thanks to Toney Allman, who sent me her excellent little book for children about Byetta and connected me with several of the Byetta users I profiled here. *From Lizard Saliva to Diabetes Drugs* (Farmington Hills, Michigan: KidHaven Press, 2006) is the only previous book dealing largely with Byetta.

Each of the successful losers on Byetta whom I profile here authorized me to quote them and to use their names. I admire their success and appreciate their contribution.

Most of this book appears here for the first time. But my Web site at www.mendosa.com, the Health Central site at www.healthcentral.com/diabetes/c/17, and five magazines— *Diabetes Health* (previously called *Diabetes Interview*), *Diabetes Digest*, *Diabetes Wellness News*, *diaTribe*, and *Type 2 Life*—previously published portions of this book in preliminary form.

Index

Bold characters indicate information in text boxes

A1C level, xiv, xx, 53
 control line of 7.0, 48
 and exenatide LAR, 18
 and individual profiles, **xxiv**,
  62, 86, 107, 132, 143, 150
 and John Dodson, 69
Abbott Laboratories, 26
Acidic fruits, 85
Actos (pioglitazone), 11, **15**, 43,
  53, **86**
Acutrim, 27
Adyvia, 29
Aerobic exercise, 67, 139–146,
  149
Albumin, 20, 21
Alcohol, **65**
Alemany, Maria, 30
Alkermes, 17
Allard, Cat, **52**
All-Bran cereal, 104
Alli, 25–26
All-you-can-eat restaurants, 129
Alpha-glucosidase inhibitors, 11,
  53
American College of Sports
  Medicine, 152

American Diabetes Association
 carbohydrate
  recommendations of, 95
 and exercise for people with
  type 1 diabetes, 141
 and fructose, 115–116
 presentation of exendin-4 at
  meeting of, 36
 scientific sessions of, 18, 20,
  21, 22, 40
 and sugar, 85, 113
 and weight training, 148, 152
*American Journal of Clinical
  Nutrition, The*, 28, 128
American Museum of Natural
  History, 32
Amylin hormone, 13
Amylin Patient Assistance
  Program, **71**
Amylin Pharmaceuticals, xx, xxiii,
  57
 and Byetta Web site, 76
 and development of exendin-
  4, 36
 and increased dosage of
  Byetta, 72–73

Amylin Pharmaceuticals,
    continued
  and launch of Byetta, 37–38
  new drugs being developed by,
    17–19
  and refrigeration of Byetta, 61
  and sales of Byetta, 13
  and Symlin, 12
Anatrim, 27
Anderson, Chris, xiii
Appetite, 4, **44**
Appetite reduction via Byetta,
    xxi–xxii, 55, 75–76, 157
  failure of with Dodson, 69
  and individual profiles, **xxiv,
    52, 111, 123**
  See also Satiety; Satiety index;
    Weight loss
Arginine, 158
Arthritis, xxii
Aspirin, 37
Atherosclerotic disease, 119–120,
    121
Atkins, Robert, 120
Atkins diet, 120, **150**
Avandia (rosiglitazone), 5, 11, **15,**
    43, 53, **132**
AVE0010, 22

Balducci, Stefano, 149
Bananas, 87
Banting, Frederick, 7, 8
Bantle, John P., 116
Barley, 85, 98, 99–101, 104
Baxter pharmaceuticals, 39
Bayer, 37
Beinborn, Martin, 56–57
Berenson, Alex, 40
Bernstein, Richard K., 139–140

Best, Charles, 7, 8
Beta cells
  dysfunction, xiv
  and GLP-1 mimetics, **44**
  growing of in patient, xii
  and type 2 diabetes, 3, **43**
Bianchi, Jean, **92**
BIM51077, 22
Bindra, Jasjit, 28
BioRexis Pharmaceutical, 22
Bison, 102, 121
Black pepper, 92
Black tea, 93
Blood glucose level, xx, 48–49, **52**
  aftermeal testing of, xiv
  control of by Symlin, 13
  and exercise, 140, 149, 151
  and fiber, 103
  and gastroparesis, 54
  and GLP-1 mimetics, **44**
  and individual profiles, **xxiv,
    39, 47, 63, 111, 123, 150**
  and John Dodson, 69
  lowering of in Mendosa with
    Byetta, xxii, xxiii, 48–49,
    52
  and use of glycemic index,
    83–84
  See also Glycemic index
Blood pressure, xxiii
BMI. *See* Body mass index (BMI)
Bob's Red Mills Natural Foods,
    99–100
Body mass index (BMI), xix, xxiv
  calculation of, 1–2
  and cooking at home, 130
  and exercise, 149
  and fiber, 104, 105
  normal for Mendosa, xxv

Bowel regularity, 103
Bradbury, Daniel, 61
Bratman, Steven, 79
Brazil nuts, 98
Breakfast, 131
Breastfeeding women, 53
Bristol-Meyers Squibb, 10
Brofman, Lance, **132**
B vitamins, 79
Byetta (exenatide), xii, xiv, xx–xxi, **15**
   and ADA scientific sessions of
      2006, 40
   authorized for sale in U.S., xx,
      37
   average weight loss from use
      of, 157
   clinical trials of and weight
      loss, 13, 36, 37, 76, 77
   compared with exenatide
      LAR, 18
   compared with liraglutide, 20
   cost of, 25, 51, 74
   and dehydration, 61
   development of similar drugs
      to, 17–24
   dosage of, 46, 70–71, 72–74
   drugs that can be taken with,
      53
   and eating strategies, **64–65**
   failures when using, xv
   and genetic polymorphism
      and weight loss, 55–57
   how it is taken, 45–47
   how it works, 43–45
   initial shortage of product,
      38–39, 40
   launch of, 37–41
   numbers of patients using,
      40–41
   and reduction of appetite,
      xxi–xxii, 55, 75–76
   and refrigeration, 61
   side effects of, xx, 55
   and slow stomach emptying,
      54–55
   stopping use of, 57–58
   success of Mendosa using,
      xxii–xxiii
   use by those without diabetes,
      25, 51
   used primarily by people with
      type 2 diabetes, 51–53
   for weight vs. blood glucose,
      65
   who cannot use, 53–55
   works after meals, 48–49
   See also Profiles
Byetta Healthcase #44 (Rubin),
   73

Caffeine, 92, 93
Calorie Restriction (CR) diet and
    lifestyle, 77–79
Calories
   empty, 109, 110
   number needed, 81
Cannabinoid receptor blocker, **29**
Capsaicin, 92
Carbohydrates
   and Bernstein, 139
   controversy over low- or high-
      diets, 95
   and fiber, 102–103
   and glycemic index, 84–85, 88
   and satiety index, 89–90
   total quantity of vs. glycemic
      index, 86
Cardiology Clinics, 120

Carlson, Richard, 116
Carlson brand fish oil, 101
Celery, 88
Centers for Disease Control and
        Prevention (CDC), 3, 122
Central nervous system, 29, 44
Certified Diabetes Educators, 66,
        78
Chana dal, 85, 97
Chemical assays, 33
Chicken, 102, 121
Children, 2, 54
Cholesterol, 103, 110
    in diet, 119
    and fat foods, 124
    and fructose, 114–115
    overall, xxiii
    and resistance training, 149
    and trans and saturated fats,
        124
    See also HDL cholesterol;
        LDL cholesterol
Cinnamon, 93
CJC-1134, 21
CLA (conjugated linoleic acid), 28
Clinical Diabetes Technology
        meeting, 40
Clinical trials, 22–24
Clothing, xxiii–xxiv
Coca-Cola, 106
Coffee or espresso, 91–92, 93
Comi, Richard, 8–9
Compellis Pharmaceuticals, 29
Compensatory metabolic process,
        154
"Complementary Therapies
        Natural Health
        Encyclopedia, The," 79

Complete Book of Food Counts
        (Netzer), 128
ConjuChem, 21
Conjugated linoleic acid (CLA), 28
ConnectiCare, 52
Contrave, 29–30
Cooking at home, 109, 130
Corn, 98
Coronary heart disease (CHD), 120
CP404, 29
CP-945,598, 29
Curare, 105, 106

D., Karen, 23
Dairy products, 120–121, 122
Dawn phenomenon, 107
Dehydration, 61, 63
Dexatrim, 27
Dextrose, 113
Diabetes
    biological vs. lifestyle caused,
        4–5
    diagnosis of, xvii–xviii
    family history of, xi
    percentage of Americans who
        have, 25
    See also Type 1 diabetes; Type
        2 diabetes
Diabetes Care, 149
Diabetes for Dummies (Rubin),
        73, 140
Diabetes Interview (magazine), xviii
"Diabetes Update" newsletter, 73
Diagnosis of diabetes, xvii–xviii
Diet
    and calories, carbohydrates,
        and glycemic, 80
    and fatty foods, 101–102

and food log, 128
foods to avoid, 109–112
fruits, vegetables, and
    legumes, 97
grains, 98–101
hard to control, 139
and low-glycemic foods, 83–84
making sure enough is eaten,
    80–82, 159
of Mendosa, 95–108
and monitoring glycemic
    index of individual, 87–88
and nutrition greater with
    organic foods, 108
nuts and seeds, 98
organic foods, 108
salad, 98
salt, 112
and stevia vs. Splenda,
    105–108
and taste of food, **92**, 95
See also Carbohydrates;
    Cholesterol; Fatty foods
Dipeptidyl peptidase-4 inhibitors,
    14
Dodson, Rev. John L., xv, 69–74,
    131
Don't Sweat the Small Stuff
    (Carlson), 116
Dosage of Byetta, 48, 70–71,
    72–74
D-phenylalanine derivatives, 53
DPP-4 inhibitors (Dipeptidyl
    peptidase-4 inhibitors), 14
Dr. Bernstein's Diabetes Solution
    (Bernstein), 139–140
Dr. Bill Quick's Byetta Web site,
    63

Dried fruit, 97
Drugs
    for diabetes, comparative chart
        of, **15**
    for nausea, 65, 67–68
    non-diabetic for weight loss,
        25–30
    that can be taken with Byetta,
        53, 54
    and weight gain, 7–15
    See also GLP-1 mimetic drugs

"Eating Rate and Satiation,"
    125–126
Eating strategies, **64–65**
Eggs, 119
Eli Lilly, xx
    and Byetta Web site, 76
    development of exenatide
        LAR, 17–18
    and development of exendin-4,
        35
    and initial sale of insulin, 7
    and LY 548806, 21
    and sale of Byetta, 13, 36, 38
Emetrol, 67
Emispere Technologies, 22
Energy-dense foods, **64–65**, 110
Eng, John, 32–36
Erasmus, Udo, 101
Essick, Kristi, 148
Eves, Neil, 149
Excalia, 30
Exenatide, 40
    See also Byetta (exenatide)
Exenatide LAR, 17–18, 58
Exendin-4, xx, 35
    See also Byetta (exenatide)

Exendin, 34
Exercise, 84, 86–87
  aerobic, 139–146
  can be enjoyable, 144–145
  as cause for diabetes, 2
  choices for, 144
  daily time required for, 155
  how much is useful, 145–146
  medical exam prior to, 140
  and metabolism, 153–155
  numbers engaging, 153
  resistance, 147–152
  who shouldn't, 141
  See also Resistance training
Exocrine, 34
Exubera, 18–19

Family history of diabetes, xi
Farnsworth, Bob, 111
"Fast-food nation," 159
Fatigue, xiv
Fats that Heal, Fats that Kill
  (Erasmus), 101
Fatty foods, 64, 65, 86
  bad for diet, 110, 112
  good for diet, 101–102
  low glycemic but not
    satisfying, 83
  and risk of type 2 diabetes,
    122–123
  and satiety index, 89–90
  saturated, 84, 110, 119–121
  and Tracy Smith, 123
  trans fat, 84, 119–120,
    121–124
  See also Saturated fats; Trans
    fat
Feathers, Tim, 86–87
Fiber, 102–105

content of food, 86
diet, high-, 84
Fingerstick testing for diabetes, 47,
  59–60
Fitness Educators of Older Adults
  Association, 148
Flaxseed oil, 87
Flax seeds, 98
Food. See Diet
Food and Drug Administration,
  38
  and Alli, 26
  approval of Byetta only for
    people with diabetes, 51
  and approval of Symlin, 12,
    13
  and approval of weight loss
    drugs, 25, 26
  and authorization of Byetta for
    sale, xx, 13
  and clinical drug trials, 22–24
  and oats and barley and fiber,
    104
  and stevia, 106, 107
  and trans fat, 122, 124
Food and Nutrition Board of the
  Institute of Medicine, 81
Food log, 128
Ford, John, 9
"Free foods," 88, 102, 105
Fructose, 113, 114–115
  naturally occurring vs. added,
    115–117
Fruits, 97, 114, 115
  fiber from, 104
  and satiety index, 89

Gastric emptying, 44, 54, 62, 77,
  103

203

Gastrointestinal
  disease, 54–55
  side effects and Byetta and
    liraglutide, 20
Gastroparesis, 54–55
Genetics
  as cause for diabetes, 2
  polymorphism and weight loss
    from Byetta, 55–57
Gerber, Jeffry N., xxi
Gerger, Renee, 39
Gila monster (*Heloderma
    suspectum*), 31–32, 34–35,
    68, 76
Ginger, 66, 92
GlaxoSmithKline, 21, 25
GLP-1, xii
  and delay of gastric emptying
    and nausea, 62
  drug to render long-acting, 21,
    35
  exendin works on, 34, 35
  mutation or polymorphism in
    receptor for, 55–57
  stopping from working by
    DPP-4, 14
GLP-1 mimetic drugs, xii, 13,
    157, 160
  and beta cells and blood
    glucose, 44
  development of new forms of,
    17–22
  and "first-phase insulin
    response," 44
  and Gila monster, 31, 32, 68
  how they work, 43–45
  and keeping weight off, 155
  lifestyle of, 75
  monthly cost of, 25

and reduction of appetite, 44
slow digestion, 44
used by people without diabetes
    for weight loss, 25
Glucagon, 33
Glucagonlike peptide-1. *See* GLP-1
Glucophage, 10, **15**
    See also Metformin
Glucose, 113
Glycemic index, xviii, 83–89
  eating low-glycemic foods,
    88–89
  "free foods," 88, 102, 105
  and grains, 98–99
  monitoring individual, 87–88
Glyset (miglitol), 11, **15**, 43, 53
Gonzales, Carole, **143**
Grady, Denise, 136
Graham, Ginger, 40
Grains, 98–101, 104
Green tea, 93
GSK716155 (formerly Albugon),
    21
"Gut hormones," xii

Harvard Health Letter, 120
Harvard Nurses' Health Study, xxv
HDL cholesterol, xxiii, 121–122
Health Valley Foods, 96
Heart attacks, 11
Heartburn, 68, 76
Heart disease
  and diabetes, 120, 122
  and exercise, 140
  and glycemic index, 89
  and saturated fats, 119
  and trans fat, 121
  and walking, 144
Heart rate monitor, 155

High-fiber diet, 84
High-fructose corn syrup, 79, 104, 114
Hiking. *See* Walking
Hippocrates, 37
Hirsch, Jules, 154
Holt, Susanna, 89–90
Homeostasis, 153–154
Homocysteine, 79, 104
Hoodia gordonii, 27–28, 69
Hopkins, Will, 149
Hormones and radioimmunoassays, 32–33
Hot-air balloon ride, 161
Human Genome Sciences, 21
Hydrogenated vegetable oil, 122, 124
Hypnosis, 67
Hypothalamus, 77

Inefficiency
  is neat, 126, 135–137
  learning to become more, 136
Injection issues, 46, 47–48, 59–60
Innodia, 29
Institute of Medicine of the National Academy of Sciences, 122
Insulin, **15, 86**
  and beta cells of pancreas, 4
  body must produce some for Byetta to work, 52
  discovery and initial sale of, 7–8
  "first-phase response," 44
  and GLP-1 mimetics, 44
  inhaled version of, 18–19
  and Metformin, Avandia, and Actos, 43

and resistance training, 149
and storing fat and appetite suppression, 4
and sulfonylureas, 43
used with Symlin, 13
weight gain from, 8–9, 11
Insulin pens, 45
Insulin resistance, xiv, 3, 43
Insurance coverage for Byetta, **71**
Internet. *See* Web sites
Investigational New Drug application, 23
Ipsen, 22

Januvia (sitagliptin), 14, **15**
Joslin Diabetes Center, 128
Journal of Biological Chemistry, The, 34
Journal of Nutrition, Health and Aging, The, 119
Journal of the American Dietetic Association, 98
Junk food, 110

Kaiser Permanente Northwest, 8, 9–10, 11
Karolinska Institute, 33
Ketosis, 141
Kidneys and kidney disease, 53–54, 81
Knopf, Karl, 148
Kolata, Gina, 76–77, 128
Kona coffee, 27
Krauss, Ron, 128

Lactose, 113
LDL cholesterol, xxiii, 119, 121–122
Leafy vegetables, 85

Legumes, 97
Leibel, Rudolph L., 154
Lemon juice, 85
Leptin, 19
Levine, James, 136–137
Lifestyle
  and Calorie Restriction (CR),
    78
  diabetes as disease of, 3, 4–5
  of GLP-1 drugs, 75–76
Linklater, Richard, 159
Linus, 97
Lipoprotein (LDL), 105
Liraglutide, 19–20
Liver, xxii–xxiii, 44
Lizzie, 31
Long Tail, The (Anderson), xiii
Low GI Diet Revolution, The
    (Brand-Miller), 90
LY 548806, 21

Maltose, 113
Manhattan Pharmaceuticals, 30
Mateljan, George, 96
Mattila, Geri, 107
Mayo Clinic Health Letter, 133
Meals, Byetta working after,
    48–49
Meat, 121, 122
Medicare, 71
Medications, taking with Byetta,
    53, 54
Meglitinides, 12, 53
Mendosa, David, xi, xii
  and Amylin stock, 39–40
  and arginine use, 158
  and blood glucose level and
    Byetta, xxii, xxiii, 48–49,
    52

and Byetta shots, 46
contact information of,
    160–161
diagnosed with diabetes,
    xvii–xviii
diet and supplements of,
    78–80, 95–108
and eating after dinner,
    131–132, 157
first use of Byetta, xx
friendship with Dodson, 72
and hot-air balloon ride, 161
learning to be inefficient,
    136–137
making sure to eat enough,
    80–82
medical condition when
    Byetta prescribed, 53
and nausea, 63–64
not losing weight too fast, 159
and resistance training, 151
success with Byetta, xv,
    xxii–xxiii, xxv, 160
and use of metformin, 10
and walking and hiking,
    141–142, 144, 146
Web site of, xviii
weight and exercise issues of,
    xviii–xx, xxi–xxiii, 151
Merida, 26
"Metabolic cells," xii
Metabolism
  effect, and spices, teas, and
    caffeine, 92, 93
  and exercise, 153–155
  rate drop and low glycemic
    food, 84
  slows with weight loss,
    153–154

Metformin, xx, 5, 8, 53
    and insulin, 43
    introduction of, 10
    profile individuals' use of, **52**,
        62, **123**
    weight loss from, 10, 12, 157
Methoclopramide (Raglan), 68
Mexican beaded lizard (*Heloderma
        horridum*), 31, 34
Microsomal Triglyceride Transfer
        Protein or MTP blocker,
        29
Mimetics, 13
    See also GLP-1 mimetic drugs
Mindless Eating (Wansink), 126
Monnier, Louis, 48
Montgomery, John, **5**
Mortensen, John, **xxiv**
Mushrooms, poisonous, 106–107
Mutation, genetic, 55–56
Myers, Ellen Ann (Annie), **62–63**
Myers, Jeff, 108

Nastech Pharmaceuticals, 19
National Center for Chronic
        Disease Prevention and
        Health Promotion, 55
National Weight Control Registry,
        133
"Natural and Alternative
        Treatments" database, 80
"Natural Health Encyclopedia" or
        "Natural Pharmacist,
        The," 79
Nausea, 62–68, **132**
    and Byetta clinical trials, 77
    drugs for, 65, 67–68
    and exenatide LAR, 18
    and ginger, 66

and metformin, 10
    remedies for, 66–67
    as side effect of Byetta, xx, xxii,
        23, **52**, **150**
NEAT, 136
Needle phobia, 46, 47–48, 49–60
Netzer, Corinne T., 128
*New England Journal of
        Medicine, The*, and
        Avandia, 11
New Glucose Revolution, The
        (Brand-Miller), 90
*New Glucose Revolution, The:
        What Makes My Blood
        Glucose Go Up ... and
        Down?* (Brand-Miller,
        Foster-Powell, and
        Mendosa), xviii, 90
New York Times, 28, 40, 69, 136
Nissen, Steven, 11
Novo Nordisk, 19–20
Nursing mothers, 81
Nutrient-dense foods, **64–65**
Nutrition Nutrient Database, 128
Nutrition Reviews, 120
Nuts, 98

Oatmeal, 104
Obesity and overweight, 1, 3, 4–5
    percentages of Americans who
        are, 25
    See also Weight; Weight gain
Oleoyl-estrone (OE), 30
Olive oil, 87
Omega-3 fats, 101–102, 110
Orexigen Therapeutics, 29–30
Organic food, 108
Orinase (tolbutamide), 9
Osteoporosis, 81

Over-the-counter drugs (OTC),
    65, 67
Overweight. *See* Obesity and
    overweight

Pain from injection of Byetta, 47,
    60
Pancreas, 4
    See also Beta cells
Parker-Pope, Tara, 130
Partially hydrogenated vegetable
    oil, 124
Patience Assistance Program,
    Amylin, 71
PC-DAC Exendin-4, 21
Peet, Alfred, 93
Peet's Coffee, 93
Pen with cartridge containers for
    Byetta, 45, 59
Penzeys Spices, 93
Peptide hormones, 32–33
Pfizer, 22, 28, **29**
Pharmaceutical marketing, xii
PharmaIN, 20–21
Phenergan (promethazine), 68
Phentermine, 27, 69
Phenylpropanolamine (PPA), 27
Plotnikoff, Ronald, 149
Poles for walking, 142
Polymorphism, genetic, 55–57
Pork, 120
Porte, Daniel, Jr., 3, 4
Potatoes, 83, 87, 89, 97
Pramlintide, 19
Prandin (repaglinide), 12, **15**, 53
Precose (acarbose), 11, **15**, 43, 53
Pregnant women, 53, 81
Prendergast, J. Joseph, xi–xv, 157
    and Mendosa, 69, 70, 72–73

and exam before exercise, 140
and government exercise
    standards, 145
and weight loss with Byetta,
    xx–xxi
Prilosec OTC (omeprazole),
    67–68
Prochlorperazine, 68
Professional-Amateur (Pro-Am)
    joint approach, xiii
Profiles
    Bianchi, Jean, **92**
    Brofman, Lance, **132**
    Coliton, Jimm, **46–47**
    Farnsworth, Bob, **111**
    Feathers, Tim, **86–87**
    Ford, John, **9**
    Gerger, Renee, **39**
    Gonzalez, Carole, **143**
    Karen D., **23**
    Mattila, Geri, **107**
    Montgomery, John, **5**
    Mortensen, John, **xxiv**
    Myers, Ellen Ann (Annie),
        62–63
    Rouse, Frances, **115**
    Smith, Tracey, **123**
    Tronier, Jana, **150**
    Williams, Ann, 78
Protein, 80, 81–82, 89–90
Psyllium husk caps, 102
Pumpernickel bread, 99
Pumpkin seeds, 98

Quick's Byetta Web site, Dr. Bill,
    63

Radioimmunoassays, 32–33
Rebiana, 106

Refrigeration, 61
Regulatory Peptides, 56
"Resistance Training and Type 2 Diabetes" (Eves and Plotnikoff), 149
Resistance training exercise, 86, 147–152
  beginning at home, 147–148
  frequency recommendations, 151–152
  numbers engaging, 151
  and sensitivity to insulin, 149
  starting slowly, 148–149
Rethinking Thin (Kolata), 76–77, 128
Rice, 87, 97
Ricola sugar-free throat drops, 130
Rimonabant, **29**
Roche, 25, **26**
Rosenbaum, Michael, 154
Rouse, Frances, **115**
Rubin, Alan, 73, 140, 145–146
Rye, 98, 99

Salad, 85, 89, 98
Saliva, 34
Salmon, 82, **87**, 101
Salt, 86, 112
Sanofi-Aventis, 22, **29**
Sardines, 82, 102
Satiety
  and coffee or espresso, 92
  and eating slowly, 125–126
  See also Appetite reduction
Satiety index, 83, 89–90
Saturated fats, 84, 119–121
Scales, 131

Schlosser, Eric, 159
Schwartz, Michael W., 3
Science, 136
Sea-Band Sea Sickness Wristbands, 67
Season and Reese sardines, 101
Seeds, 98
Selenium, 98
Serving sizes, 127
Set-point theory, 153–154
Shoes, 141
Sleep, 133
"Smart drugs," 44
Smith, Tracey, **123**
Snacking, 130
Snowling, Neil, 149, 151
Soluble fiber, 103–104
South Africa, 27
Spectrum Spread, 121
Spices, 92–93
Spirituality, 45
Splenda, 105, 106, 108
"Stalking Byetta" (Mendosa), 72
Starlix (nateglinide), 12, **15**, **39**, 53
Star Trek, 147
Starvation set point, 153–154
Stevia, 105–108, 110
Stomach
  Byetta injections in, 46, 47–48, 60
  See also Gastric emptying
Strychnine, 106
Sucrose, 113, 114
Sugarcane juice, 114
Sugars, 113–117
  and ADA, 85
  avoiding, 79, 110

and blood glucose levels, 85
naturally occurring as fructose,
115
various names for, 113–114
Sulfonylureas, xx, 5, 8, **15**, **52**, 53,
132
introduction of, 9
and weight gain, 8, 9–10, 11
Supplements, 79–80
Sweating, 92–93
Sweeteners, nonnutrient, 110
Symlin (pramlintide), 12–13, **13**,
15
Sympathomimetics, 27

Tanner, David E., 155
Taste of food, 95
Thermogenesis, 92
Thiazolidinediones (TZDs), 11, 53
Thomsen, Mads Krogsgaard, 20
TimSlim, **86–87**
Tolbutamide, 9
Tomatoes, 88
Track3 calorie counter, 128–129
Trans fat, 84, 119–120, 121–124
Transferrin, 22
Treadmill, 137, 144
Triglyceride level, 110, 149
Tronier, Jana, **150**
Twain, Mark, xvii
Tylenol (acetaminophen), 54
Type 1 diabetes
and Byetta effectiveness,
51–52
and exercise, 141, 148
and insulin and weight gain, 8
See also Diabetes
Type 2 diabetes, xx

and beta cell function, 3, 43
and drugs and weight gain,
7–15
and insulin resistance, xiv, 43
as "lifestyle disease," 3, 4–5
luck to have weight loss drugs,
159
and overweight, 3–4
as principle users of Byetta,
51–53
and resistance training,
148–149, 151, 152
three things that help control,
139
and trans fat consumption,
122–123
See also Diabetes
TZD. *See* Thiazolidinediones

"UC Berkeley Wellness Letter,"
98
United Kingdom Prospective
Diabetes Study (UKPDS),
8, 9–10
U.S. Agency for International
Development, 116
U.S. Department of Medical
Affairs, 35
U.S. Food and Drug
Administration. *See* Food
and Drug Administration
Upjohn Company, 9
Upton Tea Imports, 93

Vegetables, 97, 114, 115
Veterans Affairs Medical Center,
32
Vinegar, 85

Virtuous circle of Byetta use, xxii, 49
Vitamins and supplements, 79–80, 108
Voltaire, 145

Waist-to-hip ratio, 104, 105
Walford, Roy and Lisa, 78
Walking, 67, 91, 140–142, **143**, 144, 146
Walking staffs and poles, 141–142
Wall Street Journal, The, 130, 148
Wansink, Brian, 126–127
Water, 141
Web sites
    of Alan Rubin, 73
    Byetta, 76, 90
    of David Mendosa, xviii
    and increased patient knowledge, xiv
    "Natural Pharmacist," 79
    Nutrition Nutrient Database, 128
    world's healthiest foods, 96
Weighing oneself, 131
Weight, and diabetes, 1–5
"Weight, Weight Don't Tell Me!" (Prendergast), 74
Weight gain
    and fats, 110
    and Prandin and Starlix, 12
    and Precose and Glyset, 11
    three stages of, xiii–xiv
    and use of insulin, 7–9
    and use of sulfonylureas, 9–10
    and use of TZDs, 11
Weight loss, xiii, xvii
    and after-dinner eating, 131–132, 157
    average with Byetta, 157
    and avoiding temptation, 129–130
    and being more inefficient, 135–137
    from Byetta in profile individuals, **xxiv, 9, 39, 46–47, 86–87, 107, 111, 115, 123, 132, 143, 150**
    on Byetta requires change of diet, 76, 160
    celebrating success of, 161
    and cooking at home, 109, 130
    DPP-4 as weight neutral, 14
    and eating at table, 126
    and eating breakfast, 131
    and eating slower, 125–126
    and food log, 128–129
    and increased awareness of what is eaten, 128
    and John Dodson, 69–70
    and leaving something on the plate, 132, **132**
    and "mindless eating," 126
    minimal from metformin, 10, 12
    motivations for, 133
    non-diabetic drugs for, 25–30
    and not eating from package, 126
    not going too fast, 80–82, 159
    and resistance training, 149
    and serving size, 127
    as side effect of Byetta, xx–xxi
    and Symlin, 10–11

and willpower, 76–77, 160
    without drugs, 158–159
Weight Watchers, **47**
Weil, Andrew, 105
Wheat bran, 104
Whole Control's Golden Barley
    Cereal, 101
Whole Foods Market, 105, 106
Williams, Ann, **78**
Willow tree, 37
Willpower, 76–77
Wired magazine, xiii

Wockhart UK, 39
Women and diet, 96
Woods, Stephen, 3

Xenical, 25, 26, **27**

Yalow, Rosalyn S., 32
Young, Andrew, 36

Zealand Pharma, 22
Zofran, 68
ZP10, 22

The Marlowe Diabetes Library
Good control is in your hands.

Marlowe Diabetes Library titles are available from online and bricks-and-mortar retailers nationally. For more information about the Marlowe Diabetes Library or any of our books or authors, visit www.marlowepub.com/diabeteslibrary or e-mail us at goodcontrol@perseusbooks.com.

The New Glucose Revolution: What Makes
My Blood Glucose Go Up . . . and Down?, 2nd Edition
Dr. Jennie Brand-Miller, Kay Foster-Powell, David Mendosa
$12.95 • Paperback

———

The First Year®—Type 2 Diabetes
An Essential Guide for the Newly Diagnosed, 2nd edition
Gretchen Becker   Foreword by Allison B. Goldfine, MD
$16.95 • Paperback

———

Prediabetes
What You Need to Know to Keep Diabetes Away
Gretchen Becker   Foreword by Allison B. Goldfine, MD
$14.95 • Paperback

———

The New Glucose Revolution for Diabetes:
The Definitive Guide to Managing Diabetes and Prediabetes
Using the Glycemic Index
Dr. Jennie Brand-Miller, Kaye Foster-Powell,
Dr. Stephen Colagiuri, Alan Barclay
$16.95 • Paperback

The New Glucose Diabetes Revolution Low GI Guide to Diabetes: The
Quick Reference Guide to Managing Diabetes Using the Glycemic
Index
Dr. Jennie Brand-Miller and Kaye Foster-Powell
with Johanna Burani
$6.95 • Paperback

———

50 Secrets of the Longest Living People with Diabetes
Sheri R. Colberg, PhD and Steven V. Edelman, MD
$14.95 • Paperback

———

The 7 Step Diabetes Fitness Plan: Living Well and Being Fit with
Diabetes, No Matter Your Weight
Sheri R. Colberg, PhD   Foreword by Anne Peters, MD
$15.95 • Paperback

———

Eating for Diabetes: A Handbook and Cookbook—With More than
125 Delicious, Nutritious Recipes to Keep You Feeling Great and Your
Blood Glucose in Check
Jane Frank
$15.95 • Paperback

———

Type 1 Diabetes: A Guide for Children, Adolescents, Young Adults—
And Their Caregivers
Ragnar Hanas, MD, PhD   Forewords by Stuart Brink, MD, and Jeff
Hitchcock
$24.95 • Paperback

———

Know Your Numbers, Outlive Your Diabetes: Five Essential Health
Factors You Can Master to Enjoy a Long
and Healthy Life
Richard A. Jackson, MD, and Amy Tenderich
$14.95 • Paperback

Insulin Pump Therapy Demystified: An Essential Guide for Everyone Pumping Insulin
Gabrielle Kaplan-Mayer   Foreword by Gary Scheiner, MS, CDE
$15.95 • Paperback

———

1,001 Tips for Living Well with Diabetes: Firsthand Advice That Really Works
Judith H. McQuown   Foreword by Harry Gruenspan, MD, PhD
$16.95 • Paperback

———

Losing Weight with Your Diabetes Medication
David Mendosa   Foreword by J. Joseph Prendergast, MD
$14.95 • Paperback

———

Diabetes on Your Own Terms
Janis Roszler, RD, CDE, LD/N
$14.95 • Paperback

———

Think Like a Pancreas: A Practical Guide to Managing Diabetes with Insulin
Gary Scheiner, MS, CDE   Foreword by Barry Goldstein, MD
$15.95 • Paperback

———

The Ultimate Guide to Accurate Carb Counting
Gary Scheiner, MS, CDE
$9.95 • Paperback

———

The Mind-Body Diabetes Revolution: A Proven New Program for Better Blood Sugar Control
Richard S. Surwit, PhD with Alisa Bauman
$14.95 • Paperback